Life Lessons
of an American Woman

Life Lessons
of an
American Woman

Caren T. Camp

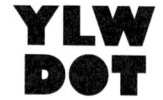

YLW DOT

©2022 Caren T. Camp
All rights reserved

ISBN 978-0-9763725-2-3

Book design by Ellen Hamilton
Edited by Vera A. Pastore, Word Choreography

No part of this publication may be reproduced or transmitted in any form or by any means, electronic or mechanical, including photocopy, recording, or any information storage and retrieval system, without permission from the author. Content relating to health and medical information is provided for information purposes only, and is not intended as medical counseling or medical advice. Readers must consult with their own doctors about any health issues they are experiencing.

Printed in the United States of America

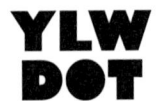

YLW DOT

Yellow Dot Publishing
Alexandria, VA 22301
yellowdotpublishing.com

Don't judge a book by its cover

Dedicated to my family of origin, the Threshies
Dedicated to my married family, the Camps

Table of Contents

Preface: Why I Wrote This Book
Introduction: Share Your Story, Change a Life

PART ONE
Finding Personal Power
1. Childhood: Setting Out on a Path
2. Careers: Gaining Independence and Confidence
3. Marriage: Maturing through Moderation
4. Building a Home: Designing on a Budget
5. Balance: Creating Realistic Expectations

PART TWO
Powering Through Problems
6. Hypoglycemia: Diagnosing and Improving
7. Adoption: Keeping an Open Mind
8. Alcoholism: Denying the Issue
9. Brain Surgery: Dealing with Trauma
10. Behavior Struggles: Loving Amid Conflict
11. TMJ: Trying Different Options
12. Back Pain: Bearing the Agony
13. Discovery: Accepting and Forgiving
14. Depression: Realizing the Depth

PART THREE
Powering Up for Health
15. Food: Opting-in on Health
16. Exercise: Varying the Routine
17. Homeopathy: Choosing Nature's Tools
18. Beauty: Protecting Your Skin and Wellbeing
19. Meditation: Calming Your Spirit
20. Pets: Adopting Canine Companions
21. Service: Applying Your Skills
22. Flexibility: Easing into the Later Years

Preface: Why I Wrote This Book

*Every experience in your life
is being orchestrated to teach you something
you need to know to move forward.*

— Brian Tracy

It wasn't until I was in my 50s that I started thinking about writing a book about the lessons I have learned throughout life. Friends would talk to me about their thoughts, feelings, and observations about the events that took place in their lives, and over the years I found myself opening up much more about sharing my own perspective. At some point along the way, I decided it would be beneficial to share my philosophy on life with people other than my immediate friends.

My parents raised me to believe that I could do, feel, and express anything that I wanted. That was a very healthy way to grow up, but there are situations and events that have happened in my 20s, 30s, 40s, and 50s that I want to share. You see, I am an American woman. I'm a product of the 1960s, I'm a product of America, I'm a product of racial prejudice, I'm a product of being a woman, and regardless of the freedom we have in this country, there are guidelines, parameters, and limitations that have affected my life. That is why I am writing this book—to pass along the lessons.

PREFACE

I feel delighted, fortunate, and grateful that I have the freedom to express my thoughts and it is satisfying to share them with others. As a child, I was taught that being a New Englander meant you ought to be stoic. In essence, show the outside world that you've got your act together, that you are happy, and that you are self-assured. Later, in my 30s and 40s, through the help of Alcoholics Anonymous and other people, I found that it was acceptable to ask for help, that it was okay to say, "I don't know the answer to this. What do you think?" I began opening up to a lot of girlfriends, other women, and therapists, and feeling more comfortable talking at AA meetings.

I thought I had my life planned at 21 but every year, every decade, I've learned new things about life and people. In this book, I want to show you that the more flexible you are, the more you will learn and the more you will enjoy life. Life changes every day and you never know what's going to happen tomorrow—you can't control it.

There is a saying in AA: "Let Go, Let God." I've relied on that guidance more and more in recent years. Nothing turns out the way you think it will. I could not have predicted the events that would take place in my life or the lessons I would learn. I have gained a lot of insight in the past six decades, and I gladly share it with you!

— Caren T. Camp

Introduction: Share Your Story, Change a Life

You are imperfect, permanently and inevitably flawed. And you are beautiful.

— Amy Bloom

Oh, that life might be perfect, right? A lofty thought, but not attainable—for anyone—regardless of gender, race, religion, level of income, education, geographic location, or career choice. Instead of reaching for a perfect life, it's more important to feel happy, healthy, and whole—doing whatever it takes to make that happen, and changing when necessary or to try something new. Maybe that's a good definition of success.

We each arrive at that point in different ways, at different times, overcoming different struggles. It may appear that other people have an easy life, but you don't know their truth. Where were you last week or last month when they were in the middle of a crisis? You were managing your own situation as well as you could at that moment. Comparing our lives to each other won't benefit anyone. Instead of comparing, share what you know!

We can learn so much from each other. Every issue, every problem comes with an infinite supply of possible solutions, some more workable than others. We have an opportunity to reach out at any moment, to find someone who may "feel our pain"

INTRODUCTION

so to speak, and gain insight from that person's experiences. Someone's hard-earned lessons can be our quick turn-around or life hack.

Passing along wisdom is a responsibility and a gift. It helps the world go around, just like love. Look at your strengths—those aspects of your personality that are second nature to you. Draw upon those strengths and your unique skills, and find someone to help. If you can make someone's path shorter or easier, do it—even if all you can offer is a hand to help or an ear to listen. When I was in my 50s, friends and colleagues started asking me questions about health, exercise, my skin care products, adoption, and other women's issues. I started journaling and realized I have learned many things in my lifetime that I want to share. I thought if I shared these things with you, it might make your life a little easier. I'm no Einstein, but perhaps the lessons I have learned as an American woman will help smooth a rough patch in your life, and maybe one day you will feel inclined to share your own wisdom.

This book is set up in three sections. In PART ONE, I clue you in to the initial chaos of my youth as well as the joy of developing a career I was passionate about and a resilient marital partnership—all of which strengthened me personally. Even though it can be difficult to divulge personal issues, I feel that I must show the early signs of problems I have

INTRODUCTION

encountered—sometimes at my own doing—and the process I used to work through those issues. So, in PART TWO, if you find yourself in any of the same or similar predicaments, know that you are not alone. Through those experiences, I found many ways to improve my health and general wellbeing, so in PART THREE I share with you information that I have found to be most beneficial. Each chapter concludes with a brief section called Life Tip to help move you forward, if that's where you're planning to go!

PART ONE

Finding Personal Power

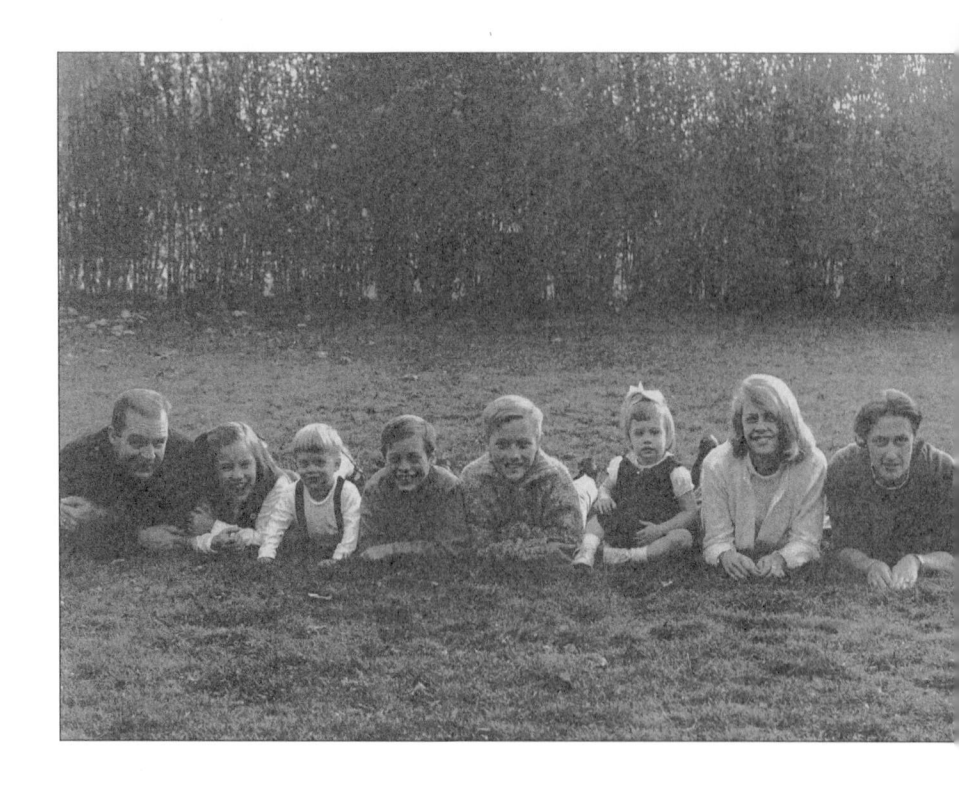

PART ONE

1. Childhood: Setting Out on a Path

One of the luckiest things that can happen to you in life is, I think, to have a happy childhood.

— Agatha Christie

I call myself "a Child of the Sixties" even though I was born in 1952. I became a teenager smack dab in the middle of the 1960s, during the Vietnam conflict, the flower child and hippie era, the birth of the "Make Love, Not War" slogan, the freedom revolution of women, the legalization of birth control, and Gloria Steinem. It was, of course, a tumultuous time and a very formative part of my life.

When I was growing up, everything in my life was extreme. I had well-functioning, alcoholic parents, we moved constantly, and when we had a party or event it was always to the extreme. We took everything to the max! My parents had six children in a twelve-year span. Three girls and three boys. I would say that my parents were great role models in a lifetime of busy-ness that included moving eleven times in the first thirteen years of my life. Those frequent moves created a lot of upheaval, but my parents never gave me the indication that there was upheaval. I felt very secure. But as the eldest, I quickly grew accustomed to having—and accepting—a certain level of responsibility that others my age probably did not experience. I was Mother's

PART ONE

right hand.

    Mom and Dad played the traditional roles of parents during the '50s and '60s. Dad climbed the corporate ladder and we moved with every promotion. My father was terrific. He did very well in business and when he came through the front door after work, we never heard a word about it. I knew he was in the textile industry with Burlington Industries but he never brought the job home. He came home from work and took over as a family man, playing baseball, kick the can, and football in the yard. He would take us on trips and relieved Mom by taking us to the circus or games and other events. He was a great dad and I remember being very happy growing up.

    I had the benefit of having an "at home" mom, cooking traditional meals and trying to juggle sports after school, homework, and birthday parties for all us kids. She was extremely creative, making custom birthday cakes and sewing beautiful handmade Christmas gifts for friends and family. And she could really craft a meal! I remember very delicious meals that we all anticipated. We got into somewhat of a routine where it would be Meatloaf Monday, Turkey Tuesday, Beef Stroganoff Wednesday, and Spaghetti Thursday. Come Sunday, she would make "Garbage Soup" that was absolutely delicious! As you might guess, it was made with the leftovers from the whole week, with no complaints. In those days, everything was homemade so there was always an aroma coming from the kitchen. There were no take-out meals and we didn't eat junk or fast food. I remember large pots of food because not only was Mom cooking for a family of eight, but many times one or more of us would have a friend over. When we asked for friends to stay for dinner, they were always welcome. A little extra water in the soup.

When I was 13 years old, we moved from North Carolina to Connecticut, as America was rebelling, evolving, and questioning. In the summers my mom would take all the kids up to Massachusetts, where we were originally from. We went to camp, learned how to sail, and learned how to eat lobsters. Summers in Massachusetts with my cousins and grandparents made for wonderful memories. Of course, the weather was much cooler and great for being outdoors all summer long.

A few years later, with the blessing of my parents, I decided to go to an all-girl boarding school called St. Mary's in Raleigh, North Carolina. I wasn't particularly comfortable in Connecticut with the drugs and the whole rebellious scene of the North, so I left. My best friend from Highpoint, North Carolina had gone there a year ahead of me. I was 16, and it was the best move I ever made because it gave me an opportunity to be an individual separate from my family. I grew from that experience and became very involved in the school. I am very proud

PART ONE

to this day that I am an alumna of St. Mary's. The private school experience taught me to be very independent and learn about different backgrounds and learning styles. I did well in school because I was comfortable adapting to new people and environments.

Looking back, I wouldn't say I had a typical, carefree childhood because as the eldest I was expected to help Mom and Dad, and that was quite a responsibility. And all that moving required a lot of adjustment but I knew nothing different. People have asked me, "How was that? What was it like to move so often?" I don't know! I adjusted, I adapted, in a manner that became second nature. I was in a new school every year or two and had to make new friends quickly. I had no problem doing that. People always say that children are resilient. Perhaps that is true because they haven't lived long enough to develop set routines, habits, and preferences, so change is easier to implement. That cycle of constant adjustment in my youth probably contributed to making me more outgoing as an adult.

One thing that I realize now is that my parents never made me feel inferior as a female. They gave me complete confidence to achieve and do anything I wanted to do from day one. The six of us had a great education, and we received encouragement and support whether we were boys or girls.

Psychologists study differences in experiences

based on order of birth in a family, such as being the oldest, the youngest, the middle child, or the only child. Growing up in the same home with the same parents doesn't make each child's experience the same. Everyone comes away with a unique perspective. For me—the oldest of six children coming of age during the 1950s and 1960s—these lessons have remained at the forefront of my mind:

- Girls are equal to boys and everybody has chores.
- Everybody in the family pitches in. No exceptions.
- Be positive. Act positive. If you can't say anything nice, don't say anything at all.
- Do not share your dirty laundry in public.
- Keep family matters within the family.
- Share, share, share—food, TV, money, clothes—anything and everything.
- Be dependable. Show up.
- Follow through with what you said you would do. Get the job done.
- Communicate. If you have problems getting the job done, ask questions.
- The faster you get the job done the better. Don't be late and don't make excuses.
- If you do the job better than what you were asked to do, you have gone above and beyond. If you only do the minimum asked, it will be considered adequate, but not great. If you want recognition or a raise

PART ONE

or promotion, go above and beyond in what was requested of you.

- Never burn your bridges. When you leave a job—voluntarily or against your wishes—always leave politely and respectfully. You never know when you will need to contact that person or company again.
- Sunday is church and family day. Anticipate that, and prepare for that.
- Look nice. Look presentable for the occasion. Dress for church in a suit, for a party in a party dress, and for school in clean clothes that are fashionable. Every day!

My Dad used to say that if you want to stay a secretary, then look like one. If you want to be an executive, then look like one, no matter your current position. If you dress in a respectable way, you will be treated with respect. I have taken this to a further degree since I lived in New York City and was in the fashion business: Look nice every time you leave the house! It's important to choose how you want to represent yourself. Even when wearing jeans, make sure they are clean, and select a nice shirt or blouse. I heard of a young woman who purged everything from her closet that didn't look perfect on her. She said, "Why would I want to look substandard?" Right.

Equipped with my childhood lessons, I went into the workforce in my 20s feeling that I could do anything that I wanted to do. Even though the nation's discussion on women's rights was just beginning, I believed that I could have motherhood and a career. Everything and anything that I wanted to do. No limitation. I wanted it all.

LIFE TIP:
Honor the lessons you gained in your youth, and add to them as you see fit. You will find that most or all of your childhood lessons continue to be valid. Learn to cook! It's a great foundation for a successful life. Be the best role model that you can be, and give your children confidence to move forward in life.

PART ONE

2. Careers: Gaining Independence and Confidence

Success is simple. Do what's right, the right way, at the right time.

— Arnold H. Glasow

People say when you want something passionately enough, the universe conspires to give it to you—someone moves out of your way or you suddenly meet an important person and that seemingly subtle act becomes the change you needed. I know this concept is true because it happened to me. But that in itself is not enough! I firmly believe you must find ways to create a good life for yourself. Set yourself up in the right location and get the right education to get where you want to go. Learn one thing, and then learn another.

I suppose I was lucky to discover my passion at a very young age. I always had an eye for fashion. I loved clothes! And I was fascinated by people in the fashion world, watching every move they made and wondering what they'd do next. I knew at an early stage that fashion—in one way or another—was my career path.

While attending high school at a boarding school in North Carolina, I took liberal arts courses but knew that fashion would be my major. By the age of 18 I applied and was accepted into a fashion merchandising school called Laboratory Institute of Merchandising (LIM) in New York City, the capital of the fashion business. All told, between the ages of 16 to 20, I had learned quite a bit "on the floor" in the retail business, working in small boutiques during the summer where I gained experience in sales and buying, and large department stores like Macy's and Alexander's. I had also done some modeling.

By the time of my graduation from LIM, I already had plenty of retailing experience and wanted to go into the field of merchandising. There were two reasons I chose to focus on merchandising. Manufacturing was the more creative end of fashion because it influenced the type of goods the retailer would be offered for purchase. Also, the manufacturing side of the industry has somewhat normal working hours—Monday through Friday from 9:00 a.m. to 6:00 p.m. Retailing had taught me that you have no personal life—just work! While my friends enjoyed the fun and freedom of staying out late, I was busy learning about working every holiday. By the time I graduated, that effort paid off because I received several excellent job offers. I chose to work for the famed Lilly Pulitzer—designer of clothing for the elite—in their children's division on 7th Avenue in Manhattan.

These choices happened naturally. Opportunities fell into my lap at different times and I caught them

PART ONE

with both hands! It felt right to choose fashion. Yes, it was my passion, but I knew that as a woman I would be comfortable in this career and would not be discriminated against, as may have been the case if I had chosen to enter another industry. I felt comfortable about my abilities in the world of fashion, I had proven myself, and I was enthusiastic about my career path.

To increase my skills even further, I decided to attend executive-level training programs with two large retailers, and by the time I was 21, I had experience in sales, marketing, buying, and management. This gave me great insight into what I did and didn't like to do in my career. I learned I had a talent in working with and managing people, and I loved working with clothing and merchandising.

During my job at Lilly, I worked with the Lilly designers, selling children's clothes designs directly to retailers. The buyers of major retailers in New York City listened to the retailers about what they were looking at from the line of children's clothes. After my first year in this position, the man running the division left and—serendipity—I took over. It was a fabulous opportunity for me.

Three years after college graduation and joining Lilly, my husband John decided to get his MBA, and we moved from New York City to Charlottesville, Virginia—an area well-known for education and history, but not fashion. I quickly found that, even if a situation is not ideal, if you truly have passion for a certain aspect of life, you can expand upon it in different ways and branch out to other related endeavors. I worked my way into three jobs during those two years in Charlottesville. I started a TV show called Fashion Today with the local NBC affiliate. This half-hour program aired after the morning news and featured fashion trends and different themes each week. It was lots of fun and a huge learning experience. Thank God the station was small enough and that I sold them on the idea and they went for it. They asked me first to raise the money to pay for the show, which I did with local retailers. That fundraising skill would prove to be very beneficial for me later as an entrepreneur. In a separate endeavor, I helped a friend establish a modeling agency in Richmond, about an hour from Charlottesville. And when an active sportswear firm opened in Charlottesville, I became the director of sales and traveled around the country and sold the line.

Then we moved to Los Angeles and I took a job with a dress manufacturer. The owner's wife was older than me and—full disclosure—hated me. She tried to make my life miserable, for whatever reason. Other than that, here's one thing I noticed while I was out there. Within an industry, there will be many similarities in the work being done, but there may also be differences due to something

PART ONE

as simple as location. In my experience, working many years on the East Coast and then suddenly heading to the West Coast, I learned that New York City fashion houses got things done immediately. The "Type A" people that I worked with in New York were professional and serious about their work, as was I. But in California, there was "mañana" attitude. That means if it gets done tomorrow or next week, cool. In New York if someone went to lunch and put a sign on the door, they would return in an hour. In California, that same sign might be there a week with no one returning.

Moving on from that experience, in 1980 I answered an ad and met a woman who was helping to distribute the newest division of Estée Lauder called Prescriptives. I was hired to help set up the new Lauder division all over the country, which meant I traveled a great deal. I would depart on Sunday evening and return home Friday night. I was responsible for hiring and training the people that would sell Prescriptives in the retailers. I trained sales people to sell the line and the correct skin care components of the line. Estée Lauder is a fabulous company and it was a terrific line.

During this time my husband had a very demanding job and we both worked hard. We talked about starting a family and thought it would be best to move back to the East Coast near our families. While living in Los Angeles we had experienced a different lifestyle, work ethic, cultures, and beliefs. After two years working with the Prescriptives line, I asked Estée Lauder if I could move east. I became a regional marketing director for Aramis—their prestigious men's fragrance line—based in Washington, D.C. I was traveling a ten-state territory and managing eight account executives. I was responsible for $10 million Profit & Loss. Lots of travel, lots of responsibility, but the move east enabled us to take our next step and begin a family.

Four months after our first son was adopted, I went back to work. The first year was extremely difficult to manage motherhood and career. Being brought up in the 1960s, I thought I could have career and family all at the same time. Some jobs can have that kind of balance. Not mine. After a year I asked Estée Lauder for a time-share situation to work part-time, sharing a full-time position with another part-timer. Unfortunately, they were not ready for that new trend in human resources, and I left Estée Lauder on good terms to stay home with our son.

We soon adopted again, and while I was home raising our two boys, I became involved in meeting planning. That's where my experience raising money for my former TV show came in handy. I joined a nonprofit as director of development to help raise money and expand their resources. As an independent meeting planner, I raised money and

PART ONE

worked with hotels and caterers, coordinating many vendors to make an event successful.

In 2001, after fourteen years at home with the children, I was ready to return to work. I joined HelmsBriscoe as a meeting planner and still love it after all these years! It suits my professional background and my lifestyle in this chapter of my life. I am not out to climb the corporate ladder or prove myself to anyone like I was earlier in my career. I like to work, I go out and find clients, and I help them with the hotel selection for their future meeting.

During my career in fashion, we did not have the Internet or cell phones. Now in the meeting planning industry, work efficiency has totally changed with all the conveniences of the wireless world. I can take my computer anywhere and therefore can work anywhere. From my past experiences I know that good customer service means listening to my clients and providing them with a service above and beyond what they could get elsewhere. That is what I strive to do. HelmsBriscoe is a company for today's times. Employees are paid commission only, so if you want to make a dollar, you better go earn it! I love to travel, and in this job, information about traveling and discovering new hotels and places is the type of knowledge that I can pass along to my clients.

I thought at age 21 I had planned my life and

career only to have it totally change two years later. Always be flexible! Do a good job! I learned that from my dad. Thinking about the ideas and energy I had back when I was peaking professionally in my 20s and 30s, I followed Dad's lessons. There was no holding me back! Dad also taught me to show up, do what you promise to do, and be dependable. These were basic rules and so easy for me to live by. I have found in my career in business that many people do not have these basic principles. Most business does not require brilliance, just follow through.

LIFE TIP:

Choose a career that will work for you in the current stage of your life—something that will fit the rhythm of your home and your family's needs. Pretend that you own the business, and consider how your role affects the success of the organization. Remember that someone is always watching, and when you least expect it, you will be rewarded.

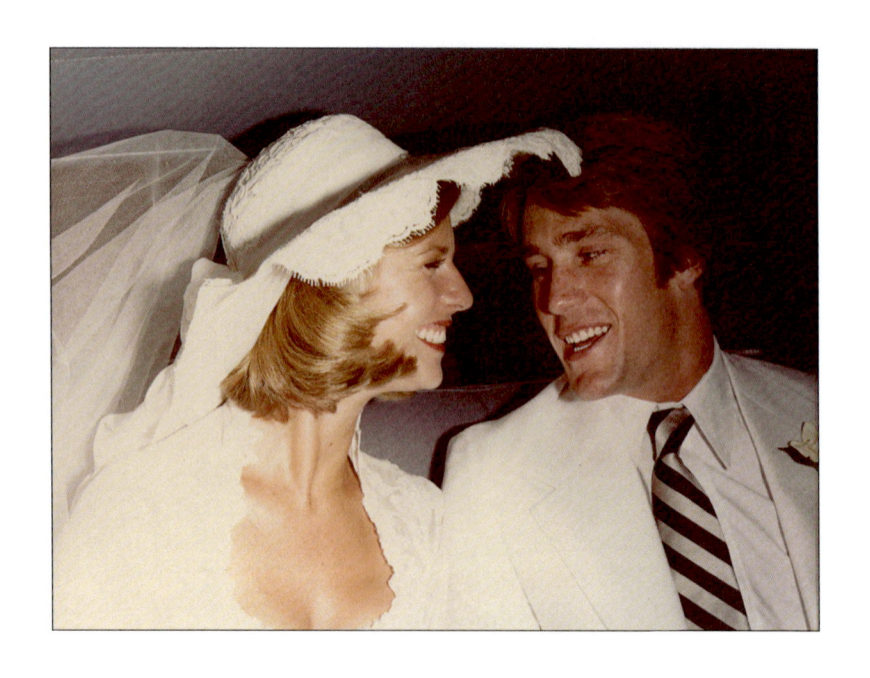

PART ONE

3. Marriage: Maturing through Moderation

A good marriage is one which allows for change and growth in the individuals and in the way they express their love.

— Pearl S. Buck

Living with John has taught me to be moderate. When we got married in 1976, I was still a drinker. There were times when he would go to sleep at midnight and I would call him a party pooper. I would stay out partying only to wake up with a hangover the next day. Later when I quit drinking, I started noticing John's moderate drinking. He would always require seven hours of sleep, he would eat three meals a day, and do things that I guess normal people do. I started realizing that living in moderation had some benefits and that I had grown up in kind of an insane environment. I learned through John—with both of us balancing childcare and careers—that living in moderation is much more pleasant.

John's a great guy, and we have learned a lot from each other over the years. I believe we have a very successful marriage. Not perfect, but it works! If you search through books on marriage, you will find variations on the themes of trust, respect, love, working together, and communication. We have done all these things and more.

PART ONE

It has not always been easy, but during the hard times we communicated. We even hired counselors who have taught us different ways to communicate and to speak to one another. We learned in a therapy session about "mirroring" that men and women speak different languages, and that different statements, questions, and comments mean different things to men and women. John and I certainly fit into that category. We learned to speak each other's language or to repeat what the other one said so we could understand more clearly what the other person felt or meant. The book, *Men Are from Mars, Women Are from Venus*, a relationship guide by John Gray, PhD, was extremely appropriate for us.

We've now been married for forty-five years! We met on a blind date in New York City when mutual friends from Raleigh, North Carolina introduced us. I knew the night that I met him—August 5, 1975—that he was a very special person. That night we played the "do you know" game, and realized we had a lot in common. We had both been to boarding schools and had a lot of mutual friends, and even had dated each other's friends. I was 22 and he was 24, and at that moment neither of us were looking for commitment or marriage. It just happened! We made plans to get together later that week. I called my mom the next day and told her I just met the man I would marry. We were engaged in nine months and married the following July.

FINDING PERSONAL POWER

    While we were dating, we talked about how we pictured our lives together, what we wanted to do with our careers, our goals, and our lifestyle. We talked about having children, our religion, how we handled our finances, whether we liked living in the city or in the country, and how we imagined growing old together. These were all issues that we thought everybody talked about before marriage. We were both fortunate that we had good role models as parents. They had been together for their lifetimes. I'm not trying to paint a rosy picture that any marriage is perfect, but if people are committed to working together, if they can complement each other rather than criticize, if they can create magic when the passion wears off, they can find ways to handle issues that will be acceptable to both parties.

    From my perspective, I think the success of our marriage can be traced to respect. I thought about that recently after a friend's visit. She commented on how John and I interacted with each other. She said she watched us first thing in the morning, preparing breakfast in the kitchen. I was feeding the dogs, and John was fixing the fruit, putting out the yogurt and the cereal. I was fixing the tea, and he was fixing the coffee. "It was like watching a ballet," she said. "Neither one of you said a word to each other, but each of you knew what the other one was doing. You would move around each other in the kitchen and it was a beautiful sight!"

PART ONE

Well, that does sound very nice! But I've only been able to learn to do this dance—and others like it—by growing in my relationship with John. By working together in moderation, it's been a much saner way to live, and it's pleasant rather than stressful. We respect each other and consistently communicate about what we do like and what we do not like. In the process of learning those likes and dislikes, we've grown to respect each other's space. I know he loves to go duck hunting and that he needs time to do that with his guy friends, and he realizes that I like to go to the beach. Time away from each other is healthy, as is understanding that the other person has individual interests outside of the couple. When we vacation, we enjoy doing many activities together, like exploring history in different countries, going to museums, and finding great restaurants, as well as hiking and whitewater rafting. We used to go running together, and switched recently to biking.

We also respect and value each other's skills and strengths, and let the other person have total autonomy over a project without interference. For example, John is very good dealing with finances and taxes, repairing what's broken around the house, and gardening and landscaping, so he runs those aspects of our lives. I am better at interior decorating and cooking, and regarding our sons, I have more patience and am better equipped to counsel them and help process emotions. He has learned to let me take the lead in these areas.

We are more similar than we are different, and this has been important in our marriage. We are both "Type A" people; we take charge and run with it. We get a job done. We do not procrastinate. In the beginning we were butting heads, but after a year, we learned to trust the other's decision and not always second-guess every action. Sometimes this compromise has required counseling. However, we have learned to step away from the other person's area of responsibility and trusted that the decision the other person made was in both our interests.

Over the years, there were times when we made mutual decisions that would benefit both of us, such as moving to new locations for job changes. And when only one of us wanted to make a change, we learned to compromise and appreciate the other's passion for making that change. For example, I instigated a few moves simply for lifestyle changes, like leaving the countryside and relocating closer to the city, and wanting to be in a better-situated neighborhood or closer to work. John was not always on board with the idea, but once we moved, he was happy about the change. Conversely, he saw a house for sale while I was out of town and told me on the phone it was perfect. I only saw it online but I could tell it was so perfect for him, and I knew I would love it. I told him to buy it before I returned.

We both loved the house.

It seems that the sharing and separating of activities, respect for our differences, and ability to compromise has worked amazingly well for us. It also helps to be best friends! We depend on each other and tell each other everything. We have remained consistent to each other and have lived up to what we agreed before we married. We also appreciate the effort we each put forth individually to manage our health, maintain a pleasing appearance, learn new things about life, and conduct ourselves professionally in our careers. When one person succeeds, both do.

LIFE TIP:

Choose the priorities in your marriage together, with input from both partners. Gather advice from other couples and marriage experts, find what works for you as a couple, and throw out the rest. Practice "dancing," and try not to settle for a two-step when you really should be doing the whole cha-cha-cha.

4. Building a Home: Designing on a Budget

Have nothing in your house that you do not know to be useful, or believe to be beautiful.

— William Morris

We weren't actually planning to build a house, we just wanted to find one that we both liked. It could have been an easy process, especially in a popular area like Northern Virginia, but it wasn't. Instead of finding the right house, though, we found a beautiful piece of land situated on a hillside in a community that we loved. An old house on the land was not worth saving so we had it removed, but we were able to keep the existing swimming pool.

Spouses may have different perspectives on how to design a home, from details like the overall size of the home to the specific features in each room, but we knew one thing for sure: we wanted to have many windows so we could enjoy the beauty of the outdoors. Having lived in California, it was important to us to find an architect who could design the house to take advantage of the views in the woods and the hillside. We ended up hiring an architect from Colorado who happened to live in Northern Virginia.

I found out early in the process of planning the design that two people cannot make all the house-building decisions together. It's impossible.

PART ONE

One person needs to be "the everyday decision maker" and the other one will be "the weekly reviewer." That's how John and I handled it and it worked fine. I was on site each day and found that daily decisions had to be made—sometimes immediately—and mistakes had to be corrected. At the end of the week, I then took major decisions to John and we discussed the best options together. He relinquished the daily involvement because he didn't have the time and he knew I would consult him on decisions important to him. I suppose there was a lot of trust involved!

We were told it would take nine months to build our custom home. As a rule of thumb, always plan on 30 percent more time and money than the contractor tells you. It's nobody's fault, generally, but unexpected things do pop up.

We realized we had to find ways to cut costs in the construction of our house because we had spent more than we planned on the land. We were going to need estimates on every aspect of the process. An architect usually costs a certain percentage of the whole project, whereas an engineer costs approximately $475 per hour. After the architectural design plan was approved, we hired an engineer to help us with the permit approvals and the questions our general contractor had. This first step saved us about $30,000.

We also identified a wood supplier. Because our lot was on a hill, it lent itself to a post and beam design. Through our search for post and beam designs, we found a business that focused on pre-engineered housing, and that offered us a service that we found very valuable. We gave the pre-engineered housing business our architectural plans and they were able to have the wood cut in the factory according to our specifications. The precut wood was shipped to the site labeled to assemble. Through this process, we saved a lot of money, and it helped eliminate the errors that are usually made on site, making the process easier. We still ended up with a custom home but saved time and money by precutting the wood. We were able to use high-quality wood like mahogany, cherry wood floors, and random width heart of pine.

One more way we saved time and money was to draw the layout of each room, marking the placement of our furniture and the location of walls, doors, and windows—even where I thought the walkways would be. This extra step helped to plan where light switches needed to be installed. Change orders are the major way a contractor makes his money once the plan has been made, so if you change walls and details once construction is under way, it will cost that much more. I avoided most of these upcharges simply by making this plan for the furniture layout. We only had one change order in our entire project.

Being home with our son allowed me to be onsite

PART ONE

every day and take part in the daily decisions. We still needed a general contractor, but between using the engineer instead of the architect and having our plans and wood precut, we saved lots of time and money. We moved into our home one year after starting construction and lived there for twenty years.

LIFE TIP:

Sometimes you just have to go big. What we wanted didn't seem to exist, so we had to create it ourselves. It doesn't always mean it will be easy or fast or less expensive, but it is possible. You can make things happen in your life, starting out with a foundation of passion and the desire to build something beautiful that you can enjoy for a long time.

5. Balance: Setting Realistic Expectations

If you want to conquer the anxiety of life, live in the moment, live in the breath.

— Amit Ray

Everyone talks about wanting to find balance in their lives—work life on one side of the teeter totter and personal life on the other. Experts say follow this or that formula, read this or that book. Sorry to tell you this, but it's not that easy. You don't just find balance while you're out on a walk. It's not a lost object under a couch cushion or in the back of a closet. You must create it!

Each one of us is so different. Our lives are full of variables with an infinite number of ways to bring them all together. When someone offers suggestions to find balance in your life, know that it's on you to create your own balance.

It's important to have balance if you desire to be happy, healthy, and whole. Actively, every day, minute after minute, the combination of thousands of decisions you make will affect your balance. Choices must be made. Certain things may need to be sacrificed. You give up one activity so you can do another.

For example, let's compare money and time. Suppose you have a certain number of dollar bills. You can buy anything you want with those dollars.

PART ONE

You can choose from many different options. But once you choose and make the purchase, you can't do anything else with those particular dollars. They are gone. You have made the exchange. Same thing with the amount of minutes you have available in your day. You have many options to choose from regarding how to spend your time, and it's impossible to do two things at once or be in two places at the same time. You must pick one.

Looking back over my life, I think I worked too much, even as a teenager! I worked every summer while I was in school, beginning with babysitting when I was 13 and adding modeling onto that the next year. By age 16, I was managing a retail store in Old Greenwich, Connecticut, going into New York City with the store owners, and consulting on trends and merchandise the store needed. After high school, I got a degree in fashion merchandising in the City, still working summers and breaks. I loved working! I graduated and got a fabulous job with Lilly Pulitzer.

However, what I learned later in life is that I was surviving on the endorphin release—the energy, the hype of work, and just being super-charged all the time. Instead of paying attention to my body, I created my very own health problem, and at age 21 I learned how to use food to balance my system better. But I still didn't know how to balance life in general.

Growing up and moving eleven times in thirteen years and then moving to New York City, I was always working in dysfunction and chaos. In fact, I thrived in chaos and the more work I was given, the more challenging and exciting it was for me. I just thought that was the way people functioned, but that's how people burn out.

I had this wonderful career in the fashion business that I adored for fifteen years. I was used to accomplishing ten things in a day and was doing my part to make everything happen. I was traveling all over the country and was always late for appointments. I was late for doctor's appointments, business appointments, and personal appointments. It was like going from one chaos to the other. Then, after working for Lilly Pulitzer and Estée Lauder for many years, I decided to quit working and stayed home with our first son when he was a year old, and everything changed.

When I made that decision, I learned the value of sitting down on the floor with my son, helping him to read a book, tie his shoes, and get dressed. Those tender moments were what life was all about and I experienced firsthand what the phrase quality of life meant. It taught me to slow down and savor the moment. Instead of being frustrated that I could not, with a one-year-old, accomplish ten things in a day—whether it was empty the dishwasher, go to the grocery store, take him to a museum, have

PART ONE

lunch with a friend, whatever—I ended up realizing that I'd rather be on time, enjoy him, and get two or three things accomplished in a day. Then I could be sane at night when my husband walked through the door.

I lowered expectations of myself and felt a sense of life balance. I was enjoying the moment and it took having children to teach me that. I was a lot happier with myself when I calmed down and realized this! Instead of setting my expectations too high and disappointing myself, I decided to set my expectations realistically so that I wasn't beating myself over the head all the time. I could enjoy my life! I was home with my children, had a successful marriage, and was able to treasure the moments. It was in my mid-30s that I really found that life balance, and it was wonderful. Years later, when I went back to work, I continued to bring that thought process into my new career. The goal was to avoid overscheduling myself or forcing too much into one day.

It helped that I was married to John, who was quite happy with moderation. I came from dysfunction, but the Camps were happy doing things moderately. I learned from watching and living with John that moderation is normalcy—not living excessively. Leave a party at a reasonable time. Sleep seven hours. Eat one plate of food, not two! Happiness is living a steady pace. No need to over-schedule with ten appointments in one day!

When I returned to work after staying home with the boys, I found a job that would fit into my lifestyle. HelmsBriscoe is a meeting planning company where I can work in my office as little or as much as I want. I have time to fit family and meals into my day. I schedule my workouts. I love working and being productive but I schedule just one or two appointments per day with plenty of travel time so I'm not late. It makes my life flow so much better and healthier!

Setting realistic expectations is a great way to guarantee some balance in your life, and I'd like to take that concept a step further and say if you really want to live in balance, expect the unexpected! Let's look at it as staying on an even keel—no matter what. Enjoy the pleasures of life, deal with the odd problems, and blend the two. Mathematically, that is:

PLEASURES + PRESSURES = REAL LIFE

Expect that unexpected situations will happen, and that you will deal with it at that point. In any given year, we all will have problems—minor or major or both. No one is immune to it. So instead of feeling panic, build time into your mental calendar to deal with problems that suddenly pop up. Then when something happens, it won't throw you completely off balance. You make the phone calls, make the appointments, ask friends for help, cancel anything that isn't important, and rearrange your schedule to allow time to handle the problem. For example, regardless if you drive a Ford or a Mercedes, there are a certain number of times each year that you will need preventive maintenance and service repairs. When your tires lose tread or your battery gives up after four years, you can say to yourself, "Okay, I was expecting this."

Now in what I call the fourth chapter of my life, I have a very nice balance of work, family, and play. So, the way I see it, balance in life relates to choosing how to spend each minute, being realistic about your choices, and recognizing that you are equipped to handle any problem that you encounter on the playground of life.

LIFE TIP:

If you are attempting to find balance, make a decision to begin life anew and ask yourself some tough questions. Are you working long hours, missing important events, feeling too exhausted to socialize or spend time with family? Are you ignoring your own needs and not allowing yourself time to recuperate from stresses? You may be able to make changes in your current job or find something more suitable to your family's schedule, or maybe you just need to cancel some activity that isn't necessary. Pay attention to your body and how you feel. Pain is the body's way of compensating for a problem. Look into it and figure out how to fix it. Avoid procrastinating, which is easier said than done, but it adds anxiety to your life and doesn't help at all. Get rid of unnecessary clutter in your home and in your mind. It only slows you down. Be free! Honor your emotions. They are real. Live your truth!

PART TWO

PART TWO

🙰

Powering through Problems

PART TWO

6. Hypoglycemia: Diagnosing and Improving

Food is not just calories; it's information. It actually contains messages that connect to every cell in the body.

— Dr. Mark Hyman

Blood sugar, as it turns out, is a thing. And we don't really find out about it until it has gone wrong. When I moved to New York City in the 1970s I was eating all the wrong things. I went to work every morning in a mad dash, grabbing coffee and Danish for breakfast. I started noticing in mid-afternoon that I would have a huge sinking feeling. I was also having sugar cravings, especially chocolate, so the afternoon slump was a good excuse to have a candy bar. When I went out at night, I was smoking cigarettes and drinking too much alcohol.

My doctor tested me, and at the ripe old age of 21, I found out that I had hypoglycemia, which is low blood sugar. I was determined not to live the rest of my life with this problem, so I started changing my bad habits and that decision transformed my life. My doctor immediately suggested that I should start eating three meals a day with protein, and it would be even better if I had six small meals with protein. While making these changes, I also decided to give up coffee.

Back then, in the 1970s, Americans had started to

become more aware of food and nutrition. I started reading a revolutionary new book called *Diet for a Small Planet* by Frances Moore Lappé about eating well to change your life. I learned what was in our food and how food fueled—or didn't fuel—the body. That book really inspired me.

I started eating three meals a day with protein, and in between breakfast, lunch, and dinner I would have some sort of protein snack like almonds, yogurt, or peanut butter. Amazingly, I felt better within two weeks. I had more energy, I didn't have the afternoon slump, and I didn't crave chocolate anymore. I decided to become a student of nutrition and learn more about the ingredients in our food.

From that experience, I became more aware of carbohydrates and protein. I learned about the dangers of eating processed foods, white flour, butter, and sugar. Even though my doctor said to eat three meals a day with protein, I became extremely disgusted with what's in American meat, so I gave up red meat. I haven't eaten red meat in over forty years. I continued to eat turkey and chicken for about ten more years and then I finally gave that up when I realized I didn't even like it. I was only eating it to accommodate others when I was entertaining or dining out. I started eating many more varieties of vegetables and other sources of protein, like beans, nuts, yogurt, and dairy products. I became healthier and more satisfied and much more

PART TWO

creative in my diet.

When I was diagnosed with hypoglycemia, I was extremely disappointed and thought that I would suffer with this diagnosis for the rest of my life. The silver lining is that it has helped me live a healthier life by making me aware of my diet and the importance of making wise choices at every meal. I'm very glad I gave up meat and switched to mostly fish for protein.

I also learned about not combining certain foods. For instance, combining protein and carbohydrates at the same meal makes it more difficult for the body to digest. I try not to combine fruits at a meal where I just had lots of vegetables.

I still eat three regular meals a day and two snacks in between when I'm hungry. I always carry raw almonds in my purse in case I get that sinking feeling and to hold me over until the next meal. I make sure I eat some protein at every meal but I don't overdo it. I learned that the reason Americans are plagued with so much osteoporosis is because we overeat protein. We don't need eggs for breakfast, turkey for lunch, and a steak for dinner. I mostly prefer vegetables and fruit, with a small amount of protein at every meal. My hypoglycemia is under control and I feel very healthy and happy!

LIFE TIP:

If you are like most people, you probably don't have all the time in the world to read every book about solving health problems through nutrition, but kudos to you if you have a personal assistant who is willing to help you with that. Otherwise, skim through several options at your local library or bookstore until you find an author who seems to speak directly to you, providing information that resonates with you. It's not about "being on a diet to lose weight." It's about becoming healthy, it's about living more vibrantly, perhaps allowing you to add more time in your life to do all the activities you are planning!

PART TWO

7. Adoption: Keeping an Open Mind

Adopting one child won't change the world; but for that one child, the world will change.

— Unknown

John and I were married for four years when we decided to begin a family. It became clear that we were going to need help, and for several years we tried infertility treatments and in vitro fertilization. It was a frustrating time for both of us, emotionally and physically, and my hormonal instincts to have a baby were raging. But we were determined to have children.

Those treatment options were not successful, so we took the next logical step and started the process to file for adoption, working with three different agencies. It is a very labor-intensive process to adopt what they call in America a "white healthy infant," which means no birth defects. These are the most sought-after children to adopt in this country, so the waiting list is typically longer than to adopt a child with physical defects or learning disabilities. We wanted a white child because we are both white, and we wanted an infant versus an older child because we wanted to bond with the baby from day one. We put down a huge deposit with each agency and waited for the phone to ring.

Prospective adoptive parents go through a tedious process of paperwork, physical examinations, financial evaluations, and psychological evaluations. My husband and I both had jobs, and the agencies wanted to make sure that our income flow would continue, despite a requirement that one of us would need to stay home to raise the child.

The wait seemed forever, but in three years we adopted a baby boy through the Catholic Charities Center for Adoption. He was born July 6, 1985 and we adopted him at twenty-eight days old. Catholic Charities told us the medical profile of the birth parents, who were age 16 and 17. They both wanted the chance to continue their education and felt that giving their baby to loving adoptive parents who were unable to conceive their own children would be the best decision. The birth mother wanted him to be raised in a Christian environment and she didn't mind that we were Episcopalian, not Catholic. Many birth mothers choose the profile of the adoptive parents, and it can be quite intimidating, being looked at under a microscope.

About a year after we adopted our son Webb, we decided to start trying for another child, and I returned to the in vitro fertilization clinic. I saw so many women go through the experience of sonograms and the tears and frustration of infertility, so I wrote an article for the doctor's newsletter about the satisfaction of adoption. I received many phone calls after it was published and I spoke to women about their frustrations. I was glad to help, since I had firsthand experience.

Unfortunately, in vitro was unsuccessful for us again and we contacted Catholic Charities to begin the process for our second adoption. After waiting a year, we were told that most birth mothers were choosing Catholic adoptive families, which meant we were in for a long wait. At this point, I learned that several of my friends were trying private adoptions instead of using an agency. To adopt privately, you place an ad in the newspaper looking for a birth mother, set up a separate phone line just for the adoption process, and hire a private attorney. So, we did that. I screened people over the phone and one day we met a woman who agreed to give us her baby when she delivered. She was about four months pregnant and we bonded with excitement immediately. I bought her maternity clothes and we agreed to pay her medical expenses.

About this time, one of my friends was going through the adoption process. She had paid for nine months of the birth mother's medical expenses and brought the baby girl home. She was given a baby shower, named the child, and had the child christened. In Virginia, a birth mother has thirty days to change her mind, and on day twenty-nine, the birth mother called and said she wanted the baby back. I can't tell you how extremely emotional and damaging this is to experience.

After that heartbreak with my friend, the birth mother I had an agreement with suffered a miscarriage. I decided I couldn't continue with the private adoption process. It was like being on an emotional roller coaster of waiting, waiting, waiting, hoping, hoping, hoping, and utter disappointment.

Next, we found an agency in Florida called Friends of Children. We weren't new to the process of adoption, but we learned there are different types of adoptions in America. A black and white adoption is very clear, with established legal parameters and expectations for both parties. A grey market adoption, on the other hand, means there are variables in the process, and perhaps, as we found, there is room for unscrupulous transactions.

In 1990, Friends of Children matched me up with a birth mother whose physical characteristics were similar to mine—tall, blond hair, and blue eyes. I wasn't aware that we had been matched during the pregnancy. When the baby was born on April 2, they contacted us and four days later we flew to Florida to pick up our son, Bob.

Out-of-state adoptions fall under the Interstate Compact on the Placement of Children, so I had to stay in Florida for ten days to make sure all of the paperwork was filed correctly between Florida and Virginia. It was a complicated process. While I was still in Florida, I learned that the birth mother had returned to the hospital for post-delivery complications, which meant I had to pay additional expenses. I asked to see the medical bill and it was astronomical, in my opinion, because we had already paid for the adoption.

   When we got back to Virginia, we had a private attorney helping us with the birth certificate and final medical records to complete the adoption. We were told that the agency in Florida required additional money in order to give us the birth certificate. We did not pay that fee for a long time, while pursuing our legal rights with our attorney.

   Bob was growing and blossoming in our home, and it felt like we were being held hostage for the birth certificate. After holding up the legal process for a year, we finally had to pay the additional $25,000, over the original cost of the adoption, just so we could get the birth certificate. There was no way around it. This agency has since gone out of business.

   Adopting my two sons has been a very fulfilling part of my life because it enabled us to unite and form a family. As they grew, we had a normal, loving relationship, but there are extra sensitivities involved for adopted children. Webb, our oldest, has been in contact with his birth parents and we have all met, but Bob still seems to be struggling with his adoption. We have been to many therapists with him over the years and have read many books to improve how we communicate.

One book I found to be extremely helpful is *Twenty Things Adopted Kids Wish Their Adoptive Parents Knew*, written by Sherrie Eldridge, a doctor who was adopted. I thought that if you adopted an infant and loved the child from day one that there wouldn't be any psychological issues. This book points out why I was wrong. It talks about the child's sense of loss for being given away and problems associated with the lack of family resemblance and differences in behavior. Many of these psychological issues come up when adopted children enter their teenage years and they are going through an identity crisis, seeking out who they are, bucking the system with their adoptive parents.

My children are adults now, and I continue reading and learning and loving. Despite the long and emotional adoption process, if I had to do it all over again, I would. That is just how special my two sons are to me. I can't imagine my life without them.

LIFE TIP:

For anyone considering adopting, I suggest filing with more than one agency because it can reduce your wait time considerably. As with any situation dealing with legal matters, do your research on every aspect of the process. Check the integrity of the agency and lawyer. Talk to other parents who are beginning the process and parents who have completed the process, and freely share information. Read books about the intricacies of relationships

PART TWO

between adoptive parents and adopted children. Keep in mind that some adoptions can appear to be happy and without conflict, but it's possible that adoptive parents may not be aware of the subconscious shadow that is said to sometimes follow adoptive children. As adoptive parents, we need to be patient, expect and honor a sudden sensitivity, and allow space for division, communication, and understanding.

8. Alcoholism: Denying the Issue

Tomorrow is the most important thing in life. Comes into us at midnight very clean. It's perfect when it arrives and it puts itself in our hands. It hopes we've learned something from yesterday.

— John Wayne

Gin and tonic. That was my first drink and I remember it well. I was 15 years old. I had fun while I was drunk but the next day was horrendous. Hung over, very sick. I'll never forget it and I never drank gin again.

After that I realized that I really liked drinking. I didn't always have to get drunk but as the years went on, I liked drinking more and more. I learned to control it around friends and family until my late 20s or early 30s, when suddenly it was controlling me. I had to drink every day. But I would wake up in the morning and say, "I am going to the gym, I'm going to work out, and I'm not going to drink today." And then an excuse would cause me to drink. Five o'clock, six o'clock, I couldn't wait until the cocktail hour rolled around. I would look for a party to go to or someone who would drink with me.

One night I had a big scare. My husband John and I lived an hour outside of Washington, D.C. Driving separately from different locations, we went to a party in the city and stayed several hours. I drank

PART TWO

too much, but we had two cars there so I drove home, following John. I got pulled over by a police officer for reckless driving. The officer looked on my record and saw I had no prior incidents. He said, "If your husband was not here to drive you home, I would put you in jail." That really scared me. At that point I really started controlling how much I would drink before driving.

Then we adopted Webb, our first child. I was 33, and for the first couple of years of his life I remember thinking I didn't want him to be influenced by my drinking. I had to control my drinking so he wouldn't see me drunk. We had worked so hard to adopt him, and I didn't want alcohol to be the main focus of our family's social life like it was when I was growing up. My parents always had cocktail parties and dinners where alcohol was the star, and I did not want to repeat that social experience for our son.

We already knew from medical records that it was part of Webb's family history—his birth father's brother had been an admitted alcoholic at the age of 18. And it was everywhere in my family. My mother was a recovering alcoholic, and my father was probably still an active alcoholic. I also had several siblings who were alcoholics. My maternal grandmother drank her whole life and was told at the age of 70 that she had cirrhosis of the liver.

Clearly there was a problem in my bloodline. I

had been to Al-Anon meetings for family members and was starting to learn the lingo—co-dependency, Al-Anon, AA. But I didn't want to believe that I also was a victim of alcoholism. I was in denial.

When I started hiding how much I was drinking from my husband, I realized I had a serious problem. He might have thought I was on one, or two, or three glasses of wine or beer and I was really on five, six, or seven, and I was waking up with hangovers. I would go to the gym, sweat it out, feel better by ten o'clock, and tell myself I wasn't going to drink that day, and again by five or six o'clock I had every reason in the world why I needed a drink.

At the age of 37 in 1990, I decided to quit drinking. It was a very hard decision—one of the hardest I've ever had to make in my life. John and I took a vacation to Palm Springs, California, and I decided that during our vacation I would tell him that I was an alcoholic (as if he didn't already know!) and that I would quit drinking. One morning he went out to play tennis and I stayed in bed, and when he came back, he said, "What are you still doing in bed? Are you okay?" I confessed what I had been hiding. I told him that I had to quit drinking, that alcohol was ruling my life, and it was very hard but today was going to be my last drink. He was incredibly supportive and wonderful and said all the right things. That night we went out to dinner. I had a few drinks, we had a bottle of wine, and then I

PART TWO

think I finished it off with a glass of champagne in a hot tub. And that was my last drink—March 3, 1990. I am now over thirty years sober and a very grateful recovering alcoholic!

One month after I quit drinking, we adopted our son Bob. I believe that God waited for me to quit drinking for Bob to come into our lives because Bob gave me such a focus. Caring for a brand-new baby was incredibly therapeutic. It was remarkable to be sober and have a new child.

My first two years of sobriety were not easy. I did go to AA, but I never had to go to a twenty-eight-day program. Thank God that I had what is called a very high bottom. For the first year, I thought about alcohol every day but I didn't crave it. I was glad that I quit. It was a huge relief. By going to AA meetings, getting a sponsor, and talking to other people in the program, I learned that they had done it—they became sober. It was a very strong, supportive program. Six months into my sobriety John and I took a fabulous trip to Italy. It was very hard to be on a European vacation with the Camp family and not drink. I considered drinking wine and then coming back and starting all over again, but I didn't. That was probably the hardest test in the beginning of my sobriety.

By the second year I found that I was dealing with a lot of emotional issues that I had covered up because of alcohol. I not only went to AA meetings but I sought out a therapist who was educated in the program, which is extremely important for anyone thinking about getting sober. There are many contraindications about alcoholism and familial roles that are extremely important for a therapist to know. I'm a perfect example—my grandmother, parents, and siblings grew up in dysfunctional environments. Though it was a wonderfully fun family, it was dysfunctional, so in that second year I came face to face with the emotions that I previously blew off. There were a lot of tears and a lot of therapy while exploring those issues, and John was extremely supportive. He went to some Al-Anon meetings and we went to therapy together, and I made it through.

I'm extremely grateful because I'm a much healthier person today—mentally and physically. My husband and friends still drink, we have a bar in our house, and it doesn't bother me at all. At parties, people say to me, "Oh, you drink cranberry and soda, why don't you drink alcohol?" Depending on how well I know the person, I say I've given it up or I have alcoholism in my family and wanted to give it up. It's not a big deal but some people really want to talk about it. Sometimes I feel they want to open up and tell me about their families or how much someone drank and it's usually a cover for their own problems or issues.

Because I have worked the program, I've been

PART TWO

much more capable of helping people. I helped two women—married with children—go through detox in my first five or six years of sobriety. One had ended up in jail and she called me when she got out, and the other one just had a breakdown. I was extremely glad to be there for them and that they could reach out to me when they decided to get sober.

When I first started attending AA meetings, I chose a location twenty minutes away from the community where I lived. I was afraid to run into someone I knew in McLean, Virginia, so I drove out to Reston. It took a few years but I eventually realized that it would be much more comfortable to go to local meetings because if I saw someone, it meant we were in the same boat, and meeting another recovering alcoholic is a wonderful gift. But in the beginning, I was embarrassed and shy about admission, and now I am not—obviously I am telling you this in a book. I am proud of it! Alcoholism is nothing to be ashamed of. It is something that affects one out of three people—a child, a spouse, a relative, a friend, or yourself. It should be discussed openly. As we have raised our adopted children, we have taken opportunities to talk about my recovery. It has made for a very healthy, open conversation, and it has raised their awareness of the illness. I am a very grateful recovering alcoholic.

POWERING THROUGH PROBLEMS

LIFE TIP:

People hide things. We do it to protect ourselves from someone's gaze, from someone's pointed finger. It's easier to believe that we don't have demons, that we're fine. We trudge along, not dealing with it, thinking of it as an asset because it is ours and we own it, rather than as a liability because it owns us. A certain amount of time passes until we realize that we can benefit by making a change. My personal hope is that everyone who decides to make a change will have a strong support system in place—whether it's one person or several—who will extend a hand instead of pointing a finger. If you recognize that alcoholism is one of your issues, gather the support and take the first step.

PART TWO

9. Brain Surgery: Dealing with Trauma

You just do it. You force yourself to get up. You force yourself to put one foot before the other and you refuse to let it get to you. You fight. You cry. Then you go about the business of living. That's how I've done it. There's no other way.

— Elizabeth Taylor

Our son Webb came into our family a few days before turning a month old. We were ecstatic, of course, especially after many years of hoping to become pregnant on our own with the help of fertility treatments, and then working our way through the adoption process. We were proud parents—the proudest!—and we watched everything our son did with glee. Developmentally, Webb progressed normally—walking, talking, and reaching all of the appropriate medical benchmarks. From a very young age, it was clear to see that his desire for knowledge was enormous. When he was around 12, I promised him I would buy any book he wanted as long as he would read it. Within four to five years of this promise, I had to sit him down and gently explain that we couldn't keep up with his book collection. It was at this point we got him his own library membership.

Since his early years he has always loved dinosaurs and managed to memorize a large majority of them. After his dinosaur years, it was onto space and wanting to become an astronaut. We wanted to support his love of space so we sent him to space camp for three summers in Huntsville, Alabama. The next phase was the FBI, CIA, and NSA . . . followed by the one thing that seems to have stuck—microbiology and infectious diseases.

By the age of 5, we knew that his intellect was ahead of schedule, but noticed that his motor skills seemed like they were lagging behind. He was not climbing like other boys and his energy levels were not as high relative to other children his age. When we would put him in a car seat, he would fall asleep immediately, as he did on a bike or anywhere he didn't have to use his own legs.

I started taking him to physical therapy, and for two years we were doing regular exercises and seeing a PT specialist. By that time our son Bob had been born. He had some unusual motor skills so we were taking him to a pediatric neurologist, Dr. John Unruh, near Philadelphia, Pennsylvania.

One day I decided to make an appointment for Webb to see Dr. Unruh also. He did some simple exercises with Webb, then laid his hands on top of his head. He told me to schedule a skull X-ray immediately. The diagnosis was craniosynostosis. In this particular condition the sutures of his skull (that separate each cranial plate) were prematurely fused together before the brain was fully formed.

PART TWO

Dr. Unruh referred us to Dr. Ben Carson at Johns Hopkins Hospital in Baltimore.

Webb was 7 years old by this time and in 2nd grade. Dr. Carson saw Webb and told me to get him on his surgical schedule ASAP. With every day that passed without corrective surgery, Webb's skull was restricting his brain from expanding and being able to grow as the rest of him did. Craniosynostosis should have been diagnosed before age 2 but had been missed by the pediatrician.

In November, 1992, Webb was admitted to Johns Hopkins for skull surgery. Dr. Carson asked us to sign a waiver alerting us to the possibility of losing Webb during the surgery. This was a level of trauma I had not dealt with before. I was totally unprepared but we had no choice. Webb needed the surgery. I was with him as he went into the surgical room and saw his head placed between braces. I held his hand, trying to be cheerful as I left. Even though we planned for the surgery, it was horrifying to see the tools that were going to cut my son's head open.

During the surgery, John and I passed the time in the waiting room the best we could. I had books and other things to read, but it was difficult to focus on the words. I would read a paragraph over and over, not retaining any of it. One of the doctor's assistants came out to say that everything was going as planned.

Dr. Carson later told me he opened up Webb's

skull from the upper front of the skull all the way back to the rear, then from temple to temple. Once his skull was opened Dr. Carson allowed his brain to expand for thirty minutes, watching it blow up like a balloon. This step was necessary because for the past seven years, Webb's brain had been restricted within his own non-expanding skull. Normally a child's cranium is soft and will grow with the brain, as long as the child is born with their sutures open. If we had not done the surgery, we were told that by age 12 or 13 he would stop walking and talking and eventually die. The surgery, which included inserting seventy-two screws to hold the skull, lasted fourteen hours. The cosmetic surgeon put his head back together, aligning skin and hair as much as possible.

After surgery Webb was taken into intensive care where he spent the night. His head was wrapped in white gauze from his forehead to the back of his head. He would drift in and out of consciousness and was able to talk and express his feelings. His eyes were alert, which was a good sign, and Dr. Carson told me that the surgery went as well as expected. I stayed by Webb's side in intensive care the whole night, and after twenty-four hours he was well enough to be moved to a regular room.

In the nine days that followed, I stayed on a cot next to him. John would come and go with food and jokes and treats. I had a friend who lived in

PART TWO

Baltimore and I would go to her house for a shower or a nap occasionally when John was there, but I wanted to be next to Webb every minute of every night and day. One night Webb woke up and said, "Mom, I can't see." It was one o'clock in the morning and his eyes were swollen shut. I gave him Arnica, and his eyes were open by the time the doctor came through in the morning. Arnica Montana is a homeopathic remedy used for swelling and pain that can be used along with traditional pharmaceutical products. Dr. Carson said Webb's swelling following surgery was the least he had ever seen.

Being in the children's ward for over a week was a traumatic experience. Children in cribs and little beds were crying at all different times. They had cancer and other illnesses that were far more serious medically than Webb's situation, and their parents were not able to stay with them. I knew that we would be able to leave the hospital in a few days with Webb because his surgery was successful, but the outcome for the others was not so bright.

Webb stayed home for three months while I homeschooled him. His head healed well and he eventually returned to 2nd grade. At the age of 15, though, some of the screws had grown uncomfortable and migrated to the outside of his cranial plates. I took him in for what we thought would be one hour of minor surgery to remove and reposition the screws. The surgery turned out to be three hours and he lost a lot of blood. The doctor smoothed out the skull and today Webb is a healthy, smart, and fully functioning young man. We are grateful for every doctor, nurse, and team member that helped save our son through all of his surgeries.

LIFE TIP:

With every illness or medical condition we encounter, we become wiser about the amazing miracle called the human body. It may be scary, especially when it's happening to your child. Allow yourself to panic for a moment, and then pull yourself together because your child needs you as an advocate to get through the process. Cooperate with the medical staff, and consider yourself as a valuable member of the team because you know many details about your child that they don't know. It's a partnership.

PART TWO

10. Behavior Struggles: Loving Amid Conflict

The children who need love the most will always ask for it in the most unloving ways.

— Russell Barkley

A young woman in Florida had a baby boy on April 2, 1990. She was tall and blonde like me, college-educated, and employed as a dental hygienist. She had been in a relationship with a guy who she did not intend to marry. She didn't want to keep the baby and made the decision to give him up for adoption.

I got the call on a Thursday afternoon and John, Webb, and I flew down to Florida the next day to pick him up at the adoption agency. We were thrilled to be able to bring another child into our home. Bob was just four days old when we met him. I stayed at my cousin's house in Florida for ten days waiting for the required interstate compact (there is a time limit) to take an adopted baby across state lines. My mother flew down from Connecticut and helped me. Bob was not taking formula very easily. Unfortunately, we did not receive much in the way of medical history because the birth mother did not wish to provide any identifying characteristics about the baby's father, so we weren't fully aware of allergies and other useful information. We tried many different types of formula before his stomach was happy accepting a nondairy, non-soy formula. I was able to bring him home to Virginia at two weeks old.

    Bob was an adorable baby full of smiles, blue eyes and blonde hair, and he was very happy until five o'clock in the afternoon when the colic set in. Then the next few hours were full of tears. Colic is a common digestive issue for newborns, generally lasting about three or four months. A few months after handling that problem, we noticed that Bob began scooting instead of crawling. Sitting up with his legs crossed in front of him, he would put both hands on the floor and scoot himself forward like a monkey. I knew right away that this was a red flag, a developmental problem, and started consulting professionals about his motor development. With the doctor's explanation and help we did physical therapy at home to help him with his motor development skills. His language skills were fine, it was just his motor development that was awkward.

    As Bob grew into his toddler phase, we would enjoy moments of sweetness with his help, full participation, and cooperation, and everything seemed normal. Then all of a sudden, he would have temper tantrums, fights, and meltdowns. This behavior resulted in many timeouts. One moment Bob would want to please and the next do something he knew was wrong behind my back or even to my face. It appeared that he knew right from wrong and did

PART TWO

wrong anyway. It became clear that he was experiencing severe mood swings and acts of defiance.

Before we knew it, it was time for school, along with an entirely new set of problems. For first grade, Bob was in a public school with approximately twenty-five children in his classroom. By the end of that year, the teacher told me that Bob needed a smaller environment where the teacher would have more hands-on time with him. In other words, more supervision. By second grade we had him in a private school with a smaller classroom and much more one-on-one with the teacher. By third grade we had enrolled him in a private, developmentally assisted school environment. I found myself at the school once or twice a week talking to the teachers about Bob's ADHD, auditory functioning, behavioral issues, and educational challenges. We hired tutors and started daily medication to help him focus on his educational classes and environment. He would sometimes hide the medicine (Ritalin or Adderall) and not take it, which only made matters worse because the medicine is intended to be taken consistently in order to control ADHD.

At age 10, Bob stole my credit card, went into the family room in the middle of the night, and used my computer to order an X-rated magazine. We had no idea that he was capable of doing something like this and he told us that he had learned how to do it from a boy in school. At this stage we were operating as if we were a police state in our own house. We were setting daily limits, restrictions, and penalties; providing rewards for Bob; and locking up things like money and credit cards. The arguments, the fights over homework, the control over food, control over taking vitamins and pills was a constant daily battle. It was exhausting to have to restrict him, monitor time outs, and enforce penalties. There were still some moments of enjoyment, love and hugging, and reading together but there was a lot of tension.

Three years later, Bob was doing poorly in school and he didn't care. We didn't know how to help him control his behavior or manage his school work. He would not talk honestly about his issues or feelings. I knew that he needed an environment that focused on education and experience that catered to children with similar challenges. We hired an educational consultant, who advised us to send him to a boarding school where they would become the police state and we could become the parents again. We took that advice and sent Bob to Cardigan Mountain School in New Hampshire. That was a good decision for him and for us. At Cardigan, Bob enjoyed sports and played soccer and basketball. He wanted to please the coaches who were also his teachers. He seemed to respect the teachers and the structure. He did fairly well for two years until six weeks before graduation. He came home for spring

PART TWO

break and filled some water bottles with alcohol and took them in his suitcase back to school. John and I got the call on Easter Sunday about what he had done. We drove up to Cardigan to pick him up because he was dismissed from the school. My disappointment and his were palpable all the way home in the car for eight hours.

    The school was wonderful working with us. They allowed Bob to finish his classwork at home, using tutors, so he could graduate and get his diploma from middle school. With the advice of the educational consultant, we next enrolled him in Trinity Pawling in New York State, which lasted only six months. At winter break, he refused to go back to school. John and I were desperate. Up to this point we had tried to include Bob in decisions concerning his school and activities, but this direct opposition caused us to adopt a more stringent approach. We didn't know what to do with Bob or how to manage his refusal to go to school and his constant rebellion. We would try to talk to him alone and with counselors to no avail. With the advice of the headmaster at Trinity Pawling and the educational consultant we decided to send Bob to a wilderness therapy program in the mountains of North Carolina called SUWS. This was one of the hardest decisions I've ever had to make.

    In order to get him to SUWS, we were advised not to tell him what we were planning. SUWS contracted with a licensed service that would pick up the incoming students and deliver them to SUWS. At two o'clock in the morning—in the middle of the night—two huge men came to pick him up. We let them in the house and we were told to take a walk around the neighborhood. They went upstairs to Bob's room and got him up. We were allowed in the room for a moment to tell him we loved him and that this was for his own good and he would be safe. They drove him away with only the clothes on his back. This was the hardest night of my life. Although it was rough, I knew it was the right thing to do for him and us. They called us the next morning and told us he had arrived safely at SUWS in North Carolina.

In this wilderness program, students live on a measured amount of food, in the woods, with counselors and other boys. Bob did not have access to any technology. Students learn to depend on their group for survival. There was daily counseling with PhD-level counselors and the other boys in the group. The boys talked about their issues and shared their stories with counselor intervention. At night everyone sleeps outside and the counselors gather up the boys' boots so they won't run away. Bob did very well because of his love of the outdoors. He was good at making fires and hiking, and he loved to sleep outside. Due to the fact that he became comfortable with the counselors and the group, Bob

PART TWO

started sharing his problems and issues.

With the help of the counselors and the administration at SUWS, they told us what type of school Bob would need to finish his high school courses. John and I visited and interviewed several schools around the country. After ten weeks at SUWS, Bob was admitted to Summit Prep in Kalispell, Montana. Summit is a therapeutic boarding school where he would finish high school while receiving extensive structured therapy. Summit had lots of structure, lots of positive reinforcement classes, and weekly counseling with other boys who were in the same situation. He reacted well to a reward system so that if he completed his work or a challenge at school, he would be able to go skiing that weekend or do some other activity. We had looked at other schools but most of them were punitive, where Summit was reward-based. We felt this option was more positive for Bob's situation.

The Summit system proved to be very successful for him. Along with individual counseling and group counseling with the other boys, Bob became much more verbal about his personal challenges with school and personal relationships. John and I would travel out to Montana every six weeks for long weekends of time together and counseling. He was not allowed off the campus or to come home until he reached a certain academic level and an acceptable level of honesty with his counselors and peer group. Once Bob reached 18 years of age, he could have left Summit, but he stayed on six more months to graduate. His choice. He graduated from Summit in June, 2000.

He came home to our house in Alexandria with a code of conduct and an expectations contract between us. In the contract we had stated what he would do at home to continue with his education and work part-time. The contract included the type of meals that he would eat, daily exercise, classes at the local community college, and part-time jobs. Unfortunately, he did not live up to the contract. The contract did not work. He started and quit or was fired from jobs in restaurants, and started and stopped classes at the community college. He was lying to us about where he was working or going to school. He could not be trusted. This cycle of lying was extremely frustrating and caused incredible tension in our home, which then caused stress in our marriage. When we asked him why he signed and wrote the contract, he said he did it to get out of Summit. We endured fifteen months of this behavior.

He stole my credit card at age 21 and charged an overnight hotel and huge bar bills, buying drinks for his buddies at a local restaurant. I finally called the police. John and Webb had been encouraging me to turn him in due to the lies, deception, thefts, disruption, and chaos. I finally had had it. The policeman

PART TWO

who came to arrest Bob was like an angel coming through our door. He told me he had seen numerous boys like Bob, including his own brother who his parents had kicked out at age 19. The policeman also told me to prepare myself for about five or six more years of this behavior. He said that once the frontal lobe development kicked in, he would mature. The policeman said during his 19 years on the force he had seen many boys like Bob at 19 to 23 years of age. Then as they entered into their late 20s maturity would set in. Eventually, we would see this start to happen around age 26 to 27 for our son. He took Bob off to jail. I will never forget that policeman's words. I visited Bob in jail a few times. He told me that he learned a lot because the other guys in jail could see that he was privileged and advised him "to get his ass out of jail" and grow up. Ultimately, I think it was a great learning experience for him.

Each year I prayed that Bob would turn himself around, find his way, and make it through without hurting himself or someone else. And learn something, which he has.

During the time when Bob was living with us, we would experience moments of both sweetness and anger. I so enjoyed the days when he was thoughtful in the kitchen helping me with cooking or setting the table. Each time he would challenge my patience I continued to pray the sweetness would win out in the end.

Finally, after living at home for a year and not doing what he had promised he would do, we had to kick him out. We constantly tried and suggested he have counseling. I realized he was telling the counselor what he or she wanted to hear. When we finally found a counselor who saw right through him and challenged his lies, he didn't want to go to that counselor anymore. Then I would challenge him and arguments would go around in circles.

We kicked him out and he became homeless for nine months, traveling around the country with three other people. He would go into libraries to email me, letting me know how he was or where he was. I was glad to know that he was alive. He told us later that he had "worked the system." He and his friends had begged on corners for money, slept in homeless shelters, and jumped trains. Played music for money. Got beaten up in Chicago.

One beautiful day in October, I was on the Eastern shore of Maryland at our house after doing a bike ride. As I drove home, Bob and his three buddies showed up on our porch. I was so excited to see him! Gave him a hug and welcomed them all into our home. They were all filthy because they had been living in the same clothes for nine months. Fortunately, we had an outside shower. I gave them all clean clothes and washed theirs. I fed them for three days and listened to their stories about living on the streets and jumping trains! Wow, was I glad

PART TWO

he was home safely. After three days they all took off to North Carolina. One week later I got a call from Bob from New Orleans. He was ready to come home for good. Could I send him a bus ticket? I did and he made it home.

There were times when it seemed that he was so troubled that I became very scared for his life. He was reckless, and didn't seem to care if he hurt himself or anyone else. While he was living with roommates in Arlington, Virginia, Bob would hole himself up in his room and not respond to anyone. He didn't eat. Sometimes he would take food from his roommates at night. He could not function to go to work. I found him living in months' worth of filth—with boxes from pizza and empty soda cans all over the floor. He would not let me in his room, and seemed not to care to live. I couldn't see a clear path forward for my son who I loved so much. I didn't know what else to do or where to turn. I wondered if he was feeling suicidal. Out of desperation, I took Bob to his favorite counselor at Summit Prep in Montana. He diagnosed Bob as bipolar. Bob accepted the diagnosis and started on medicine. After a year he stopped the meds.

At this point he was 23 years old. He would have a restaurant job for eight or nine months, then something would happen and he would move. It was constant upheaval. Not only would he change jobs but he would get kicked out of a roommate situation, either due to not paying rent or lying or stealing. He went through four or five jobs in a three-year period. Then in July, 2017 he was invited to a wedding in Asheville, North Carolina. While he was there, he called me and said he was moving to Asheville. That it is his kind of town. Artsy, casual, cheaper than Northern Virginia. And he felt he had a better opportunity to succeed there.

So, he moved. And he met a girl. He's still happy there. And making an honest living.

Each year I've seen more maturity in his conversation about his jobs and his life. He takes responsibility and has stopped blaming others for things that go wrong. He is happier. He has a job and a home and a girl.

What advice do I have for others raising a Bob?
- Love your child. Provide positive reinforcement when your child makes good decisions.
- Patience. Count to ten or twenty before losing your temper.
- The Internet offers a huge amount of temptations and resources. Wade through the information and find what makes the most sense for your family's situation.
- Hire a professional, like an educational counselor.
- Listen to the teachers, the school, and the professionals. They have all seen these personalities before.
- Do not set your child up for failure. Establish some

perspective on what the child can or can't handle regarding school, living situations, and work.
- Don't put your child in a situation where failure will be the path of least resistance.
- Establish limits and expectations. And hold firmly to them.
- Try to instill morals, expectations, limits, and ethics, and hope that those lessons last and eventually come through.
- For a young child, create a reward structure for accomplishing small tasks, like getting ready for school or completing homework. Receiving a certain number of stars on a chart can result in a reward each week or month.
- Have faith in the research that maturity will develop in the mid-20s.

LIFE TIP:

As parents, we love our children and we want the best for them. We want their lives to be better than our own childhood may have been. We want them to experience success, happiness, and prosperity. It's not always easy, and there are no guarantees. Every child comes with a unique set of circumstances, characteristics, and challenges. Parents are the role models, the providers, the doers, the ones with more experience and the wisdom to start and end each day with love.

11. TMJ: Trying Different Options

Some days are better; some days are worse. Look for the blessing instead of the curse. Be positive, stay strong, and get enough rest. You can't do it all, but you can do your best.

— Doe Zantamata

As a child, my teeth were fairly straight and I didn't need braces. But in my 20s, my dentist in New York City said that one of my front incisors was starting to stick out. He suggested braces and I did not want that. So, as an alternative, he shaved off my teeth on one side in order to make room to push the incisors back into place, while I wore a retainer at night.

It worked but I did not know that shaving teeth can change the whole dynamic of a person's bite. Teeth have electrical currents that run up and down from the upper teeth to the lower, so it's important that the teeth are lined up in the correct place in the jaw. I did not realize until much later that the electrical current was disturbed when my teeth were shaved, and that was the beginning of my jaw disorder.

Four years later, something happened to create more trouble for me. I was living in California at that time, and threw a party at my house. Apparently, I was having a great time dancing, and

PART TWO

suddenly turned a certain way, smashing my head into the edge of a door. I was taken to the hospital with blood gushing from my eyebrow. I went home with seven stitches and a huge black eye.

After this incident the headaches started, sometimes becoming migraines. The pain that went up my neck into my jaw also radiated to my right shoulder. The pain was constant and some days excruciating. Eventually the pain radiated down to my whole right side, affecting my hip, low back, and right leg, continuing down to the arch and big toe of my right foot.

I initially discussed this pain with my dentist, and two years passed before he diagnosed it as temperomandibular joint disorder, or TMJ for short. He sent me to a TMJ specialist who put braces on my upper and lower teeth. The pain got better within two weeks, so I believed this specialist for six years and went through adjustment after adjustment. I still had pain in my head and down my right side but he kept telling me it would take time to improve. I was having massages to relieve the pain and finally saw a physical therapist who alerted me that something was still very wrong.

Unfortunately, I learned that this doctor believed he could help people with TMJ but he was really making money keeping me as a patient. I found out that some dentists would attend sessions for TMJ education and then call themselves specialists. At this point I was desperate to feel better. I was in my late 30s, had two children, and was trying to function as normally as possible. I was having a rough time, but considering myself to be a strong woman in America, I continued to power through the way I always had.

After investing eight years in "fixing" my jaw, it still was not right. I wanted a second opinion, and in the summer of 1993, I found out about a dentist in St. Louis, Missouri, named Dr. Jim Jecman. He also had a degree in osteopathy, which means he knew how to feel the muscles in the neck and back, what position they were in, and whether or not they should be moved. He explained that when he used braces to move teeth, it would affect the patient's neck, spine, and back. He could not move teeth effectively without taking into consideration how it would affect the rest of the body.

When I first saw Dr. Jecman, he put a new set of braces on my teeth. Then, with me on a table, he adjusted my neck and back for almost an hour, performing gentle manipulations. I flew from Virginia to St. Louis every month for two years while he successfully adjusted my braces, my back, and my neck, putting all the pieces back in alignment. I credit Dr. Jecman with saving my life.

When I finally got the braces off in my early 40s, I had no more headaches and no neck pain, but I still had pain in the right hip. I found out about eight months later that my hip pain would be another chapter of my life. But my TMJ was gone. It had taken ten years to solve and correct.

LIFE TIP:

    Regardless of a doctor's pedigree, some doctors are wiser than others, in the same way that some accountants, lawyers, and hair stylists are wiser than others. If you are dealing with a serious physical issue, get a second or third opinion and educate yourself so you can ask intelligent questions to help solve the problem. Track the symptoms and be able to provide details. The body is a master puzzle, and every piece needs to connect in order to reveal the whole picture. Finding the corners is just the beginning.

12. Back Pain: Bearing the Agony

There is no coming to consciousness without pain.

— Carl Jung

People typically associate suicidal tendencies with emotional disorders, but I struggled with those thoughts at a time when I was experiencing severe physical pain. The pain in my back and hip was so excruciating that it was hard to function, and there were days that I just kept thinking—how can I live like this?

During the years that I had TMJ treatment on my jaw, I was constantly told that the reason for my back and hip pain was due to my jaw being out of whack. I accepted this story and lived with the pain for years. When I finally got my TMJ fixed—surprise—I still had hip pain. I pursued a doctor and found that, with traditional X-rays where the patient is standing or lying down, the spine is flat and certain types of problems don't show up. This doctor had me do a flexion X-ray where I stood bent over, and he saw the disc that was protruding from my lower spine—the L5–S1, which carries the most weight and is most prone to injury. In this condition, called spondylolisthesis, the protruding disc is usually pinching a nerve called the sciatica. That sciatica pain traveled fiercely down my leg.

In December, 1999, I had a fusion in my lower

PART TWO

back that fixed the spondylolisthesis. The surgery was successful, and soon I was doing physical therapy. I was in much better shape than before the surgery, but I was not out of pain. I will always remember this conversation with the physical therapist:

"When will I be relieved from this pain that I am still experiencing?"

"Probably never."

"What do you mean by that?"

"Most people who have back surgery will continue to have some sort of pain."

I reacted the same way anyone would have reacted—I burst into tears. A few months later I returned to my surgeon at Johns Hopkins Hospital in Maryland for a follow-up visit. The fusion in my lower spine looked good and healthy. It lined up and was holding, so he considered the surgery a success. I was so anxious to have this condition fixed, that I guess I did not ask enough questions prior to surgery. What I didn't know before, and didn't find out until after, is that most back surgeries will create another sort of pain because it cuts through numerous muscles in the back. It can affect the patient permanently, as it has me.

Knowing what I know now, would I have that back surgery again? Yes, because it eliminated about 75 percent of my pain and I no longer thought of looking for a way out. Since then, I've learned through physical therapy, massage therapy, osteopathy, and all the exercises and stretches that I do, that I'm going to have to live with pain almost every day. Some days are worse than others.

Looking back on the situation, I wish I had known in advance to lower my expectations. I thought surgery would solve my problem, but it really only decreased the problem. I didn't know the pain would last forever. Fortunately, through a lot of self-discipline and a little bit of patience, I have found that a variety of physical activity and exercise helps to keep me moving, comfortable, and functional.

Here is what I do to combat the pain:
- **Lacrosse ball.** I use a lacrosse ball to alleviate the spasms in my buttocks caused by my piriformis muscle—the large muscle that runs through the buttocks.

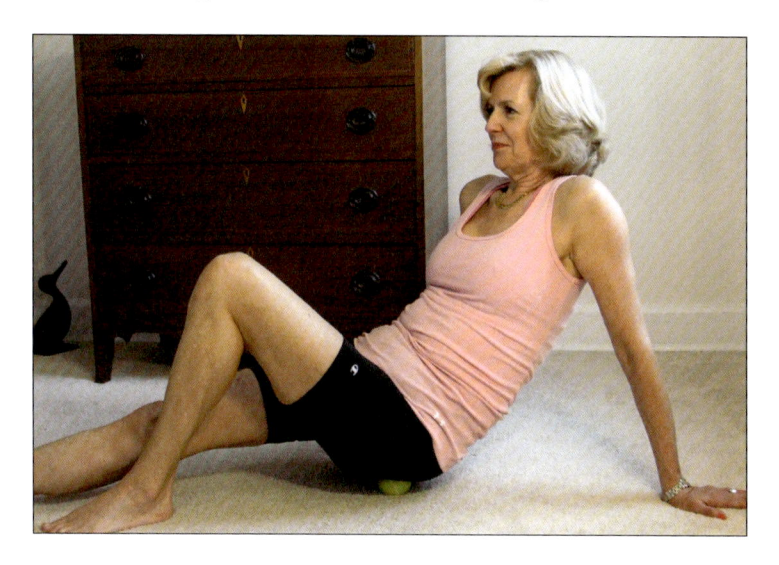

I roll on the ball, back and forth and up and down. It is extremely invasive, but it is the hardness and specific shape of the lacrosse ball that allows the piriformis to release.

- **Ice pack.** While sitting at my desk, watching TV, or having dinner, I put the ice pack on my lower back or hip for ten or fifteen minutes. It helps to alleviate the pain and take the swelling of the muscles down. This helps a great deal.

- **Resistance band.** While lying flat on the floor, I place the band around the arch of my foot. Holding onto the ends of the band, I raise my leg straight up above my head, pointing to the ceiling, then over my right shoulder and over my left shoulder. I hold each position for fifteen seconds to stretch my hamstrings.

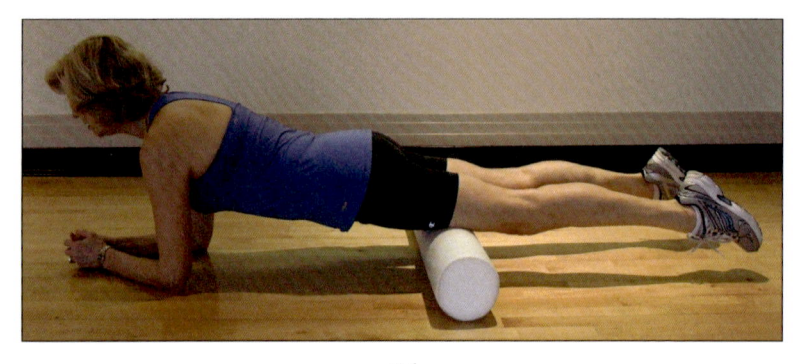

- **Foam roller.** To release the tension in my lower back, I use a Styrofoam-type roller that is about five feet long, similar to a pool noodle float but denser. It's been extremely helpful in relaxing my back, gluteus maximus, hips, and hamstrings, especially at the end of the day. It loosens knots and breaks up adhesions, providing a deep tissue massage. While on the floor, I hold my head up and roll my lower back up and down, up and down on the roller. It usually gets the snap, crackle, pop. On the days that my hips and hamstrings are tight, I also roll back and forth on my gluteus maximus and hips. Then I raise one leg above the other, put all the body weight of one hamstring on the roller, use my arms to prop myself up, and roll up and down on my hamstring. It's very effective. I also use the roller lengthwise from my head to my tail to open up my chest and shoulders.

- **Clock circle.** The most effective set of stretches and toning exercises I do for my lower back doesn't require any equipment. On my back, I rock my hips (left hip, right hip) from side to side about ten times, isolating each hip bone one at a time, pointing up to the ceiling separately. Then I rock my belly button and pelvis towards the ceiling (front to back, front to back), again isolating each one towards the ceiling. Then in a circular motion I do a clockwise rotation of my hips, my back, and each hip separately rolled into the floor so that the other side is elevated, followed by a counterclockwise rotation. When I do this rotation, I sometimes feel the crunch in a particular spot on my back. It's good to roll slowly through that spot until it is smoother. Sometimes that requires coming back to that spot many times to help it release. These stretches are extremely effective for loosening up the pain at the end of the day, as well as for stabilization of my lower pelvis and spine.

PART TWO

It sounds like a lot, doesn't it? But all of these activities probably take less than ten minutes in the evening before I go to sleep, and the benefit far outweighs the investment of time. When I travel, I always take the lacrosse ball, the Pilates circle, and the exercise band. The sciatica pain running down my leg is the most intense, so I will roll on the ball every night, no matter where I am, to loosen up the piriformis muscle and relax the sciatica.

LIFE TIP:

Many people say to rely on surgery as a last resort. Do whatever you and your doctor think will provide the most benefit. Learn as much as you can about the physical body—before something goes wrong—and do your best to give your body what it needs. Get the proper nutrition and exercise, keeping in mind that your needs may be different than others' needs. Address what ails you and keep it moving!

13. Discovery: Accepting and Forgiving

You either get bitter or you get better. It's that simple. You either take what has been dealt to you and allow it to make you a better person, or you allow it to tear you down. The choice does not belong to fate, it belongs to you.

— Josh Shipp

Adoption records through Catholic Charities are closed. We knew the profile of our son Webb's birth parents and they knew ours, but no names or details were provided and the two parties were not to meet. One day Webb received a certified letter from his birth mother. She had spent four years tracking him down with the help of a private investigator. The letter said she had birthed a son on July 6, 1985, which she believed to be him. Webb was furious. He marched into my office and said, "How dare she give me up and then try to come back into my life 22 years later?"

He gave me the letter to read. It was beautifully written, and must have required a great deal of emotional control to write and send, not knowing how it might be received. She expressed a desire to give him medical information of herself and the birth father, only if Webb wanted to know it. She was very pleasant in her explanation and was not asking for anything in return.

PART TWO

I knew how much courage it took her to take this step. Opening yourself up—being vulnerable—is a risk that can lead to emotional trauma or newfound joy, and there is no way to predict the outcome.

Webb remained agitated about it for a year as the letter sat in his desk, without responding to it. As a mother who has adopted a child, you always wonder if someday this type of contact would take place and how it might turn out. I had prepared myself for every possible scenario. I told him it was lovely that she had offered the information, especially since he was getting older and could one day have children of his own, and medical information could be useful for many reasons.

Every once in a while, I would ask him what he thought about her letter. The following winter, just before the holiday season set in, they started emailing each other and eventually agreed to meet after the New Year. He was scared and nervous and decided to take a friend with him, which seemed like a great idea. When they met at a restaurant in Washington, D.C, they ended up talking for several hours. That night when he came home, he told me it was like meeting an old friend. I was so delighted for him! I was relieved that the meeting went so well and they both chose to let love rule rather than anger and hostility. I think their reunion boosted my son's self-esteem in ways I couldn't have anticipated.

John and I later met Webb's birth parents. They did not marry each other but both live within thirty minutes of us. We invited his birth mother to our house for Webb's 25th birthday dinner, and we shared all the pictures of his growing up years. There were tears of joy and lots of happiness. Not all meetings of adopted children and both sets of families are that successful, so we all felt blessed that everything had worked out.

Today Webb's birth mom has a family with three children. Webb and I have a very nice relationship with her. When Webb turned 30, I emailed her and said, "Thank you for the gift of his life. There could be nothing more meaningful and generous than what you did. It made our family what it is today." And she responded, "It brings me great joy to know that any tears I have now are of joy in regards to my decision thirty years ago. It was a dreaded day in that office. Who knew that what I saw and chose on paper would be so perfect for Webb? I could never regret my decision with you as his mom."

LIFE TIP:

Egos are especially fragile when dealing with a meeting of birth and adoptive parents. It may be difficult to know how to act in front of this new audience. The child is on center stage and emotions are overwhelming. In the role of adoptive mother, drop back and follow your child's lead when making decisions about meeting birth parents. It gives the

PART TWO

child a sense of having control over a major life event. Maintain a stance of patience and respect for all parties, including yourself. Hopefully everyone will bring the appropriate props to the meeting—scripts that they have rehearsed for years, baskets overflowing with love, and cameras to capture every angle.

14. Depression: Realizing the Depth

A human being can survive almost anything, as long as she sees the end in sight. But depression is so insidious, and it compounds daily, that it's impossible to ever see the end. The fog is like a cage without a key.

— Elizabeth Wurtzel

Three years after my maternal grandfather died, my grandmother basically stopped eating and drinking water. Her death certificate said she died of dehydration but she was totally depressed. She was in her 70s, and it's possible her depression had started earlier, but it didn't become obvious until her husband died. And in those days, I don't think they gave people antidepressants. She basically killed herself from depression.

My mother became sober in her early 50s, and a few years later she battled depression. It was so bad she would tell me that she would wake up in the morning and feel like there was an elephant sitting on her chest. She couldn't get out of bed, she couldn't function, and she didn't even want to get dressed or eat. Sometimes she would spend the day in her nightgown and never get anything done. Finally, doctors put her on an antidepressant. She functioned for many years until the effects began to wear off and she had to switch to another antide-

PART TWO

pressant. She ended up with three or four types of antidepressants, and it helped her immensely to be able to function.

Grandmother, mother, me. I realized that I could inherit a tendency towards depression but I had hoped to avoid this problem because I felt I had taken steps to protect my health. I had been a healthy eater since my 20s, I quit drinking when I was 37, and I incorporated various types of exercise into my life. However, at age 57, depression hit and it hit so badly that I began contemplating suicide.

Generally speaking, perhaps most people deal with depression because things aren't going well in life, but for me it was the opposite. I had a loving husband and a strong marriage, I had two children and a career, I had money in the bank and healthy food on the table, I had no alcohol in my life and a workable exercise regimen, so I felt that I had hit all the milestones. In my mind the end of my life had come. There was no reason to continue. So almost every day I would contemplate whether I was going to kill myself with a gun, a knife, or a car accident. I would go to sleep at night thinking about it, I would wake up in the morning thinking about it, and throughout the day behind the wheel of a car I would think about it.

Of course, there was the rational side of the mind saying, "You don't want to die by suicide" and the other side of the depression would say, "Yes, you do, just end it now. You're miserable, you've finished your life, you have nothing else to live for. Just finish it."

This internal debate went on for a year, and to an outsider, I was functioning. I would put on a happy face, I would put on a party face, I would put on a social face, I would put on a family face. I wasn't going to AA meetings on a regular basis and even when I did go, I only talked about controlling alcohol and not drinking, and that I felt good about my program. But I wasn't sharing depression. I had put it in this other little category in my mind and just thought, "I'm not going to address it."

One day in December, 2009 I shared it with John. I was crying. I needed to tell him goodbye and that I loved him and that I did not see any future. He said, "You're depressed. Your mother was depressed, your grandmother was depressed, and you have not been able to avoid depression. Get help."

Why was it so obvious to him and not to me? I don't know the answer to that question. I want to share this because as healthy as I thought I was, I was actually very sick. And when I saw those ads on TV that said "Depression hurts" I would think, "Oh, well, that's just marketing and advertising," and I would ignore the message. Eventually I made an appointment with my regular doctor and told her about my problem with depression. She put me on a low dose antidepressant once a day and two weeks later I was my old self again. The depression—the thought of killing myself every day—went away. I rediscovered the happiness that I used to have every day, the gratefulness. It wasn't an act; it was really me. I was glad to be alive!

LIFE TIP:

Depression exists on many levels. It may have been building up over a long period of time or may appear in the dark of night like an unexpected guest. It's wiser to address it than to ignore it and stuff it in the back of a closet you rarely use. Even when you think life is running smoothly, a bump may throw you off course. You don't need to face it on your own, but you do need to face it. Reach out to a friend, a family member, a doctor, and you can get it packed up and sent on its way.

POWERING THROUGH PROBLEMS

PART THREE

PART THREE

❧

Powering Up for Health

PART THREE

15. Food: Opting-in on Health

The body is your temple.
Keep it pure and clean for the soul to reside in.

— B.K.S. Iyengar

My family lived in many places when I was young, but there was always one constant no matter where we lived—we were always a typical meat and potatoes family. My mother was a very good cook, and made meatloaf, baked chicken, leg of lamb, and other favorites during the week, followed by a big stew with the leftovers on the weekend. Along with the meat and potatoes, we always had a salad and vegetable. But like many American families in the 1950s and 1960s, meat was the main course.

As a young adult, I went through a period of not taking care of myself—smoking, drinking, and eating unhealthy foods. I cared more about my work schedule and social calendar than my body. After being diagnosed with hypoglycemia, I turned myself around.

The first book that inspired me was *Diet for a Small Planet*, which helped me improve my health after that diagnosis. My doctor suggested having several small meals per day with protein. At this point I gave up meat and caffeine and felt better within two weeks. Later I read *Fit for Life* by Harvey and Marilyn Diamond, which was about how to eat—

POWERING UP FOR HEALTH

by paying attention to food combinations as well as timing. This concept totally changed my thoughts on food, because I never knew that one food had anything to do with another food being eaten at the same meal. But I learned that certain food combinations make the body's internal organs work harder for digestion and can cause fermentation. Another bestselling book about nutrition and health I read later is *The China Study* by T. Colin Campbell, which shows a relationship between certain types of food and chronic illnesses.

I changed not only what I ate but also how and when I ate. I continue to follow that guidance still today. I do not eat fruit after vegetables for several hours. I do not combine protein and carbohydrates. When they are combined, it makes it very hard for the body to digest.

When I was in my 30s, a friend told me about body fat and the foods that create body fat. She told me that eating a chunk or cube of cheese was like putting it right on your hip like a square of cellulite. That statement changed my eating habits. I stopped eating cheese and lost four percentage points of body fat in five months. Over the years I started using a little fat-free feta in my salads but I don't buy cheese unless it's for company.

Today I get total joy out of being a pescatarian, but most of the time I eat veggies. When I first started being vegetarian, I thought I needed to eat lots of pasta. In my 30s and 40s I ate pasta at least three or four days a week. Then 50 hit. I learned about the hazards of too many carbohydrates and I discovered better ways to get protein and vegetables. Now my lunches and dinners are filled with a salad full of raw vegetables—a variety at each meal. This represents 50 percent of the meal. Then about 10 to 15 percent is a protein such as beans, fish, tofu, soup, or veggie burger. The rest of the meal is cooked greens. Once in a while I will have a carbohydrate such as Kashi, quinoa (also a protein), pasta, brown rice (a perfect complement with beans), or a sweet potato—the most perfect nutritious food you can eat—topped with nonfat yogurt or tahini.

FAVORITE MEALS

After many years learning about food, nutrition, and health, I now rely on several favorites that work well for me. For example, twenty minutes before eating breakfast I drink Monavie (an acai berry drink) mixed with no-sugar Knudsen pure cranberry juice. I also take a probiotic capsule, which has millions of acidophilus and bifidophilus—good bacteria that are naturally found in the digestive system. These good bacteria need to be replenished.

Then for breakfast I eat one cup of low-fat cottage cheese with blueberries, strawberries, or raspberries and a few walnuts, along with homemade granola sprinkled with chia and wheat germ. I also have two cups of green tea with fresh lemon juice because it aids digestion, especially first thing in the morning. I slice a lemon in half, heat for thirty seconds in the microwave to make it easier to squeeze, and use half in each cup.

Once a week I have two poached or soft-boiled eggs with multigrain bread—my favorite is Ezekiel. Once or twice a week I have steel cut oatmeal sprinkled with walnuts and almonds along with berries and kefir, which is a liquid yogurt.

For lunch I usually have a veggie burger (no bread) and a salad of dark greens such as arugula, spinach, or kale, with carrots, celery, tomatoes, and bean sprouts. Or I may have a salad and bean or lentil soup, or salad and a piece of fish from dinner the night before. Always a salad!

A good dinner would be wild salmon, a green vegetable like broccoli, kale, spinach, or asparagus, and a salad. We always look forward to grilling Portobello mushrooms, eggplant, and other favorites every summer.

In addition to the three main meals of the day, I enjoy a mid-afternoon snack of an apple, herbal tea, or a few raw almonds or walnuts. If I'm on the go, my favorite snack is Think Thin protein bars—20 grams of protein and no sugar.

FAVORITE RECIPES

Nut Mix. I found out that roasted nuts lose half of their nutritional value, and if they are seasoned or salted it adds unnecessary sodium, so I buy raw nuts and store them in the freezer until ready to use. Then once a month I make a nut mix, storing it in the refrigerator, using raw walnuts, almonds, and pecans. I add dried cranberries, crystallized ginger, pumpkin seed, fennel seed, cinnamon, and other spices I have on hand.

Granola. I make granola once a month to use on top of yogurt and fruit for breakfast or I eat it with soy milk. It has no sugar but is delicious and high in fiber. This recipe is based on one created by the culinary team at Rancho La Puerta (www.rancholapuerta.com), with a few minor changes:

  3 cups rolled oats
  ½ cup almonds, chopped or sliced
  ½ cup sunflower seeds
  ¼ cup oat bran
  ¼ cup whole wheat pastry flour or oat flour
  1 Tablespoon cinnamon
  ¾ tsp. ginger
  ¾ tsp. cardamom
  ¾ cup honey, maple syrup, or agave syrup
  ½ cup unsweetened apple juice
  2 Tablespoons vanilla extract
  2 tsps. cold pressed oil
  2 tsps. grated orange peel
  2 Tablespoons fresh orange juice

Preheat oven to 275 degrees. Mix all ingredients in a large bowl. Place mixture on large baking sheets. Bake 35 to 45 minutes or until lightly browned, stirring several times. After cooling, store in an airtight container.

Lime Salad Dressing. I have read many articles about how we eat too much vinegar in our prepared foods and dressings. Too much vinegar can cause digestion problems and can lead to yeast infections. When I found this recipe, I started making it every month as a delicious alternative. It's so easy—mix it all together and keep it in the refrigerator!

Juice of 1 lime
½ cup olive oil
1 large garlic, minced
1 Tablespoon chopped white onion
2 tsps. fresh chopped cilantro
¼ tsp. veggie salt
¼ tsp. cayenne pepper
¼ tsp. cumin
Black pepper

LIFE TIP:

If your family wants to opt-in on health, there is much to consider. Food is complicated business! Some food is simply healthier than other food, and you have to do the research and make some choices. Everybody likes variety in their life and in their meals, so try alternating the type of vegetables you eat every day and experiment with a variety of spices to see what you like best. Invest some time to look through recipe books and find some options that call for ingredients you like. Some people like

PART THREE

to use recipes with only a few ingredients—that's fine! There are many quick and easy recipes created by other health seekers, and you are sure to find something appropriate for your family.

16. Exercise: Varying the Routine

Lack of activity destroys the good condition of every human being, while movement and methodical physical exercise save it and preserve it.

— Plato

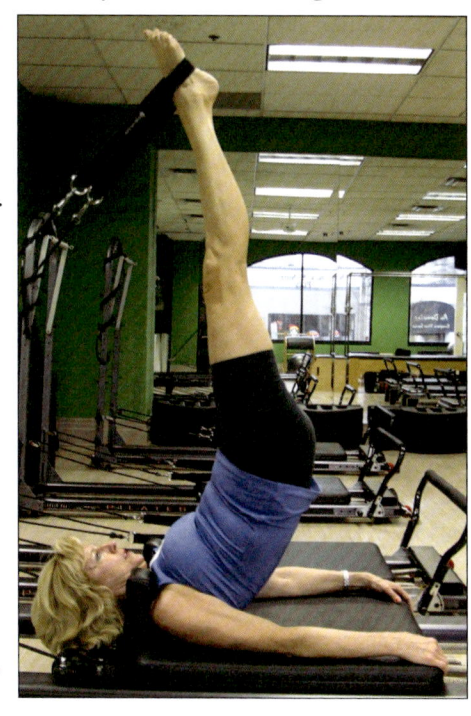

I didn't always love to exercise like I do now. When I was young, I simply wasn't interested, but it started to grow on me by playing basketball in high school. Then after college I started running and learned that I loved the release of endorphins and how exercise not only made me feel good but also helped me to stay slim. I began to plan my whole day around my running schedule. When I married John, we ran together in the morning, and when I traveled, I only stayed in hotels that had a gym (which is very easy today). I loved running through the cities early in the morning, especially San Francisco. I loved running the hills and seeing the city wake up.

Fast forward about fifteen years. I suddenly realized all that running had taken a toll on my back, hips, and knees, and I was in pain. I was only in my 30s when I needed back and knee surgery. Then I learned about the benefits of biking and using safe machines in the gym. I started using the gym regularly and hired a personal trainer who taught me about the importance of interval training and how it helps burn fat. This really changed my routine! He measured my body fat when I started, and in just a few months I had burned off several percentage points of body fat. Book coauthors Dr. Henry Lodge and Chris Crowley discuss this concept in their *Younger Next Year* series, which I highly recommend for everyone age 40 and above.

These days I have quite a routine set up so I can get some type of exercise every day. It powers me up and I feel like I'm taking positive action to maintain a healthy lifestyle. I go to the gym at least three times a week and once a week I do Pilates for flexibility and strength. I incorporate yoga stretches into my routine, and I walk my dogs daily. Biking has become my favorite aerobic activity, and I may not even consider it "exercise"—it's just fun!

At some point I suppose I decided that exercise shouldn't be considered as something that has to be done; it should already be an integral part of our day as much as flossing our teeth or combing our hair. For example, if you are a skier and you go on a ski trip, that is your exercise for the day. You shouldn't have to feel obligated to lift weights on the same day. You're done! For someone who enjoys biking, do a thirty-mile trip with the intention of having lunch at the destination. Nature lovers can take a three-hour hike while enjoying the landscape of their choice, at their own pace. There is no rush. It's not a race! Gyms have a variety of day and evening classes for bodies of all skill levels, as well as personal trainers to help fix you and challenge you.

Living with a bad hip and leg, I've learned that I must vary my workout to use different muscles each time. I have training equipment that I use at home on days I don't go to the gym—resistance bands, Pilates circle, lacrosse ball, large stability ball, weights, and a foam roller. Options, options, options!

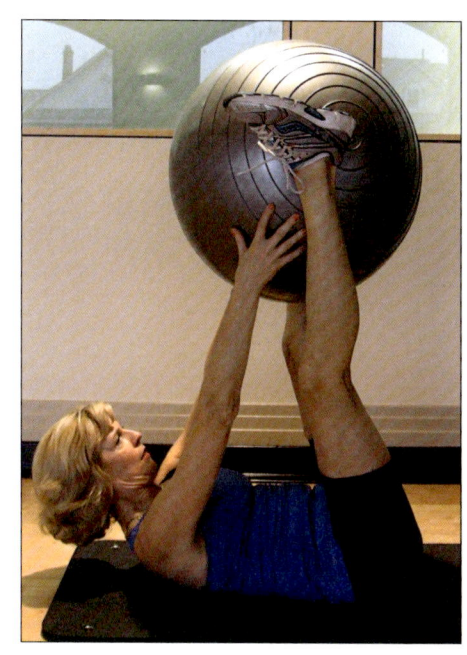

PART THREE

LIFE TIP:

If you are doing some type of exercise that you think is beneficial but causes pain, stop! Check it out with a doctor and research alternatives to relieve or eliminate the pain. If a physical therapist or personal trainer teaches you specific moves to correct a problem, follow the proper form, otherwise your effort may be wasted. There are many ways to do an exercise incorrectly. Trust the experts!

17. Homeopathy: Choosing Nature's Tools

Homeopathy cures a larger percentage of cases than any other form of treatment and is beyond doubt safer and more economical.

— Mahatma Gandhi

In my early 20s I learned that the practice of modern medicine consisted of going to the doctor to get a pill. In other words, "Take this pill, go to bed, and see if you feel better in the morning."

Fortunately, I started reading about nutrition, diet, and wellness, and I learned about an alternative approach to medicine called homeopathy that dates back to the experiments of Samuel Hahnemann in the late 1700s. He was a German physician who discovered that "like cures like"—the principle that an illness could be cured with a medicine that would actually create those same symptoms in a healthy person. Homeopathic treatments eventually became popular many years after his death, until the early 20th century when the competition of modern pharmaceutical companies put homeopathic apothecaries out of business here in the U.S.

So today we don't see a lot of homeopathic apothecaries or pharmacies in this country like there are in Europe, where you can find one on almost every corner. Many Europeans swear by the use of homeopathy, but Americans are not quite as aware

PART THREE

of its uses and benefits. Homeopathic doctors can write a prescription for an antibiotic or a medicine but their initial way to cure you is homeopathically. That was my choice, and it was important to me to delve into this option.

    I found a homeopathic doctor in Fairfax, Virginia. I also read a couple books about the subject and attended a few all-day seminars to learn which homeopathic remedy to use for various symptoms. I took my children to that doctor from the time they were infants and learned that homeopathy is extremely effective. My boys grew up with very little conventional medicine because we used homeopathy for fevers, temper tantrums, and other symptoms that were easily curable. I would say 90 percent of the time I was able to solve my children's problems, diagnose their symptoms, and make them feel better with homeopathy. To this day, they will ask me for a homeopathic remedy for any maladies they are having before they consider pharmaceutical drugs. It is my choice as well.

    For example, pine bark was the original "aspirin" used by Native American Indians and maybe also the Chinese. When you have trauma or pain to the body, you can use Arnica Montana, which contains pine bark, to help alleviate the pain. If I have overexerted myself, had a fall or an injury, I will take Arnica Montana before bedtime two or three times a week and wake up feeling much better the next day. Another example is Belladonna, which I relied on heavily for my children's fevers.

Homeopathic remedies are easy to use, have fabulous results, and are inexpensive. You will find them in health food stores, specialty grocery stores, and apothecaries. I purchased a large kit that has as many as fifty homeopathic vials in it. I have learned over the years which ones to use for different situations. They never expire and many of them are useful for traveling.

Here is a list of some of my favorite homeopathic remedies that we have used frequently:

- Arnica Montana: for pain, injury, surgical procedures, muscle strain

- Belladonna: for high fever, sunstroke

- Nux Vomica: for nausea, vomiting, indigestion

- Rhus Tox: for poison ivy, joint sprains, stiffness

- Chamomilla: for sudden fever, great irritability, restlessness

- Hepar Sulphuris: for painful boils and earaches with pus

- Pulsatilla: for colds, earaches, gastric upset from fatty foods

- Spongia Tosta: for croupy cough

LIFE TIP:

I'm not a doctor, I don't play one on TV, and I'm not dispensing medical advice here, but I can tell you that homeopathy has worked successfully for my family. We have been using it for several decades, along with conventional medicine when necessary. Learn about all the treatment options available to care for your family. Rely on the healing tools provided by nature before turning to chemicals in pharmaceutical drugs. Always consult with a homeopathic physician if you have questions about the proper remedy for a specific ailment.

18. Beauty: Protecting Your Skin and Wellbeing

People will stare, make it worth their while.

— Harry Winston

I started working for Estée Lauder in 1980 at age 28, and I'm glad I did. The cosmetics industry doesn't focus solely on beauty products—it's also about health—so having this particular job at a young age helped me to become aware of the importance of skin care and the hazards of sun damage. I was trained in a new line of skin care called Prescriptives. Through a microscope, I could see the damage to skin that had been exposed to the sun as well as skin that had no sun damage. The lasting impression had been made. I never went in the sun again without wearing a very strong SPF. Still to this day, each morning before going to the gym or walking the dogs, I apply La Roche-Posay Face SPF 50 lotion with tint.

After the little microscope incident, I immediately started to care for my skin. I started having facials once a month and began using both night and day creams. During the day I would wear a moisturizer with SPF, then a powder or base with tint and SPF.

Then I learned about Endermologie, a non-invasive deep tissue massage that treats areas prone to cellulite—hips, legs, and abdomen—using a special machine administered by a trained technician.

PART THREE

It helps to eliminate cellulite and increase blood circulation in those areas. I do this procedure once a month. Daily I use Bliss body wash in the shower with a plastic stimulator and mint scrub, and then Bliss Fat Girl Slim to firm the skin. I have been following this regimen for years and I believe that the combination of diet (not eating meat), drinking lots of water, and the Endermologie treatments is the reason I have very little cellulite.

When I got to my 40s, I made another major change and began having monthly microdermabrasion treatments—otherwise known as lunchtime facelifts, or MDA. The esthetician uses a wand with fine granular sand on the end, creating a gentle abrasive action to exfoliate the skin, and the dead cells are vacuumed away. Depending on your skin, it can be rough or smooth. This process opens up the pores and exposes the bare surface of the skin. After having one of these treatments, the skin can be pink or red for a short period of time, and you must protect it from the sun and elements carefully for at least three days. It is important to use a product that has no perfumes or harsh chemicals in it. I have come to love Agera's MagC Peptide Serum, which I now put on every night after washing and before moisturizing. It is quite pricey but I think it's worth every penny. Serums are the best, new remedy in skin care.

This microdermabrasion technique to exfoliate

and rejuvenate the skin was brought to the U.S. in 1995, a decade after it was developed in Italy. It helps to improve sun damage, wrinkles, enlarged pores, and scars, and stimulates blood and lymph circulation and the production of new skin cells. My esthetician says I have been doing these treatments for so long that my skin has become stronger and more resilient, and I believe I also have fewer lines.

   It's important to find a good esthetician who is very educated in skin care and certified to perform microdermabrasion treatments. I have gone to, and continue to go to, the same esthetician for 20 years. She is terrific and has stayed current on information about the newest products. She taught me about a wonderful line of products called Esthederm, which is only available through the best salons. I only use it at night due to its expense. The eye cream is incredible, as well as the night cream and cellular water spray.

   Another product that I get from Agera is the Vitamin C activator and mask. I use these once a week. It is a granular type of wash that keeps pores clean and only takes one minute when I'm cleansing. I have larger pores and this process helps minimize them.

   My day skin care treatment is a line from Switzerland called Arbonne. I use the Nutria C for mature skin. After cleansing I always use a spray toner (no alcohol), a day serum, eye cream, and day cream with SPF. Then I use Jane Iredale tinted SPF, which has just enough color to smooth the tone of my skin without looking like too much makeup. I also use Jane Iredale powder, applying with a brush. It has moisture in it, does not get in the lines, and has a fabulous color and coverage. Another great, but less expensive, line for mature skin is Bond No. 7 Restore & Renew night cream, day cream, serum, and eye cream, which can now be found at Target and Amazon.

Entering my late 50s, I learned about the Fraxel laser, which resurfaces the top layers of skin, and BroadBand Light therapy, which helps remove the brown spots that have accumulated from sun damage over the years. This process needs to be done in a med spa or doctor's office where a doctor has supervision. I usually do these treatments in the winter when it is easier to stay indoors for a day or two while recovering from puffiness, redness, and swelling. I do Fraxel once a year because I have been doing MDAs for so long that my skin responds very well to it. Some people may need Fraxel treatments more often.

All in all, it only takes a few minutes each day to take care of your skin. Health practitioners seem to be in agreement that drinking eight cups of water per day provides many benefits for the body, including the skin. I also drink Monavie, an acai berry concentrate, which is high in antioxidants and has helped improve my skin.

Along with managing skin care, I love using Estée Lauder makeup products, especially the lipstick. I have learned that drugstore makeup can be great if you know what to look for. I use Revlon lipstick; it has nice moisture, does not spread into fine lines, and the colors are great. I also use Revlon eye shadow and Neutrogena blush. Sephora is also a great resource. I buy the best mascara called Blinc. I have long eyelashes and mascaras always used to get smudged under my eyes. Blinc encircles each lash and stays on all day, and it doesn't smudge. It's more expensive than other mascaras but lasts for two or three months. I also use Smashbox eye shadow—great colors. When you order from Sephora you get free samples and an opportunity to try new products, and that's a wonderful way to live!

Lipstick, blush, and eye shadow—color is everything. Have you ever put on a dress and something about it didn't seem quite right? It may have been the wrong color for your skin. While I was working with the Prescriptives line years ago, I learned that my color tone is red/orange. That means my most natural makeup and clothing colors are coral and melon. For contrast, high fashion, or nighttime, I can wear pink and red. Colors I should not wear are green and yellow because they are not flattering for my color tone. Therefore, I have three sets of lipstick, blush, and eye shadow, depending on what

PART THREE

color clothing I am wearing and whether it is day or evening. I always wear lipstick and blush in the same color family, and try to use a complementary eye shadow. It's always best to wear eye shadow that complements the color of your clothing, whether warm (brown, taupe) or cool (blue, gray, black). The goal is to feel good about how you look!

LIFE TIP:

Caring about your appearance isn't vanity—it relates to good health. Physically and emotionally! Our skin has a big job to do—protecting our internal organs. But the skin itself is an organ, and our job is to protect it from all outside influences. Products and treatments that help do that are important to consider. Makeup and skin care products can be expensive, so depending on your budget, do the research and find the best options for your unique skin care needs. Perhaps the products in one line will suit you, or you may want to pick and choose items from several different lines. Looking good and feeling good helps boost your self-esteem and confidence, so I say go for it!

19. Meditation: Calming Your Spirit

While meditating we are simply seeing what the mind has been doing all along.

— Allan Look

In the 1970s, America was experiencing a period of social and environmental activism, as well as a New Age of spiritual consciousness and transformation. "Transcendental Meditation" was a very hot subject. I was living in New York City, and like most New Yorkers, I was working too hard and not eating right. I was diagnosed with hypoglycemia, which is low blood sugar due to poor nutrition. A very wise doctor gave me two suggestions: change my diet and learn how to meditate. I was feeling very poorly all the time and decided I was not going to live the rest of my life that way. I changed my diet and began learning how to do Transcendental Meditation (TM).

TM—a natural way for the mind to reach a calm state of rest—was taught by qualified trainers. Using TM as a daily practice, I found out, would provide a positive impact in many areas of physical health, including eating and sleeping habits. I went to a little office on the West Side of Manhattan and over the course of several weeks, I learned how to meditate. Meditation is not something that happens right away. You have to be able to get into a state of mind of relaxation. The trainers gave me a specific

PART THREE

mantra—a special sound or word—that would be effective to help me focus. As I was very energetic and hyper, it was a bit difficult to quiet my mind. It took me a while, but I soon learned how to meditate.

Meditation was a life-changing experience for me. I followed the regimen they taught me: meditate for twenty minutes in the morning soon after rising but before eating, and then sometime in the mid-afternoon between three and four o'clock. When I did meditate successfully and came out of my meditative trance, I felt like I had had eight hours of sleep! I was absolutely refreshed. I was calm, I could concentrate, and I could work on a project or do whatever I needed to do.

I practiced meditation for quite a few years and found it to be extremely helpful. Nowadays you can read a book about meditation, come up with your own mantra, and get into a trance for twenty minutes. I highly recommend it for anyone in any stage of life. It is a wonderful habit and there are no drawbacks.

But as in everything in life, you don't know until you know. If someone never heard of meditation or never tried it, it may be impossible for that person to see the benefit, and that's exactly what happened at the adorable little private school my son Webb attended for kindergarten. All the parents were paying top dollar for their children to be there. Mid-afternoon, the children had rest time for thirty minutes. One of the teachers, who I think was Asian, taught the students a type of meditative stance. Knowing the full value of meditation, I thought it was a wonderful option since youngsters are so full of energy—doing art projects, running around outside, and climbing on playground equipment. Thirty minutes of relaxation in the afternoon is terrific and much needed, even if all they do is lie down and stare at the ceiling.

Well, one of the parents found out that they were having relaxation time in the afternoon and complained to the Head Mistress that she wasn't paying all this money for her children to be lying down doing nothing. Unfortunately, that is the mentality of most of America. We think we always have to be actively running on full power to consider ourselves productive.

When I was meditating on a regular schedule, I actually found that I was much more productive after taking twenty or thirty minutes to relax and go into that stance. It's easy to set an alarm and find a word to focus on or go into a "happy place" zone. Sometimes I would close my eyes and imagine ocean waves breaking on the sand. It was a hypnotic image that made me feel refreshed.

When I got married to John, we were both runners. For many years we ran together, and in a way, I found it to be my meditation. At some point I stopped meditating, and after I turned 50, I decided that I needed time for meditation back in my life. I was not able to bring up my old TM mantra again after thirty years but I designed my own way of relaxation. I read that lying down and elevating the feet is a very good relaxation posture for the middle of the day. Because I live with a sore back, this is what I do. I lie down flat (no head pillow) and elevate my legs on two large pillows to make my back flat on the floor. This position also helps the blood circulation go to my head and relaxes all the back muscles. I then meditate or relax by thinking of the ocean or the most pleasant place I've ever been. I am lucky that I can do this for about twenty minutes as then I feel refreshed for the rest of the day.

LIFE TIP:

Throughout your life, you may have seen various relaxation techniques or behavioral programs that offer many health benefits. All of those techniques may be useful, but some may not resonate with you. That means a program might not fit into your schedule, it may seem too difficult, it may be outside your budget. Try several options and see what works best for you. Your best friend may love one program, and you might love another. That's okay.

20. Pets: Adopting Canine Companions

A dog is the only thing on earth that loves you more than he loves himself.

— Josh Billings

Two heads are better than one, as they say, because two people can share ideas, offer suggestions for problems, and help each other make complicated decisions. And two dogs are better than one because they can entertain each other while you are away from home. That means they'll be happier, you'll be happier, and perhaps you won't return to find the tips of your favorite shoes chewed off. Two tails waggin'—that's what you want to see!

Dogs give unconditional love and expect nothing in return, other than a bowl of food and refreshing water. They never ask for diamonds, to go to Disney World, or to paint their bedroom neon green. They might want a fenced-in yard, but they will never demand it.

Deciding to adopt a dog is one of the best choices you can make to improve your physical health and emotional wellbeing. Having a dog reduces blood pressure and stress while also boosting your mood. So much research has been done showing that people who have dogs live longer, happier, and healthier lives because they have a sense of purpose—something important to focus on other

PART THREE

than just themselves. I believe it's true. And they are wonderful for children. Not only do dogs protect and share a bond with children but chores like feeding, walking, and cleaning up messes are great lessons. Learning to take care of a dog forces children to create and follow a schedule, to be dependable and responsible, and to be held accountable for "issues"—all very important skills that carry over into other areas of life.

In forty-five years of marriage, John and I have had ten dogs—usually two or three at a time. Most of our dogs have been Labradors, which are easy-going and wonderful with children. Once we were given a Norwich terrier—Buster was a pistol with a strong and very enthusiastic personality! Dogs are very social animals and play with each other and take care of each other, but one dog alone waits for the humans to walk him, feed him, entertain him, and pay attention to him. John and I work full time so we're in and out during the day and frequently have work responsibilities out-of-town. So having more than one dog helps in many ways. Our dogs have always been awesome companions for us and for each other.

Pets, in general, and specifically dogs, become a big part of the family. Over the years, every time I have lost a dog it feels like I have lost a child. I grieve and mourn the loss, and it's tough to recover. The last time we lost a dog—Lightning—a month went by and I really did notice a huge gap in my life not having a dog. So today we have Ruby and Daisy, barking at each knock on the door, just like it says in the Pet-Human Partnership Agreement.

We love to walk Ruby and Daisy in the morning before breakfast and at night after dinner. We meet lots of wonderful people in the dog park nearby, but we don't really know their names—just their dogs' names! It's so much fun to see our dogs running around, having a good time with the other dogs. It is an incredibly positive social interaction in the community, and it's quite an experience to witness firsthand all the unconditional love the dogs give their humans.

When I think about all of our dogs—Sugar, Spice, Pepper, Thunder, Nutmeg, Bingo, Lightning, Daisy, Ruby, and Buster—I am amazed at how much our lives have been enriched. Dogs are truly like angels on earth... helping us, loving us... and reminding us of the wonders of life.

LIFE TIP:

If you are contemplating the two-dog scenario, you don't have to get two dogs at once or from the same litter. You might already have a dog. If you pair an older dog and a younger dog, the older one can teach the newbie the house rules on getting outside, how to use "inside voices," and how not to gnaw on table legs while waiting for handouts at dinnertime. Because, let's face it, not gnawing is Lesson Numero Uno!

PART THREE

21. Service: Applying Your Skills

Only a life lived for others is a life worthwhile.

— Albert Einstein

Many options exist in life: work or don't work; work here and not there; wake up early for church or sleep in; eat vegetables or sugar, fat, and salt; think only about your needs or think about others. I have read many times that taking part in some type of activity that helps others raises your endorphin levels and makes you feel better. That is certainly true for me.

I enjoy volunteering for many reasons. It provides an opportunity for me to give to others less fortunate. It makes me feel useful, like I am helping society in some small way. I feel a personal commitment to certain issues, so volunteering allows me to help those organizations meet their goals of serving a specific population. It also gives me a chance to get involved in my community, make important decisions, and meet some really amazing people.

For many years I have served on boards where I can get involved in projects to raise money and then help decide where that money will be spent. Through CASE, the Center for Adoption Support and Education, I raised money for adoption counseling; through the Ethos organization, I helped with drug and alcohol addiction treatment and prevention; and for ACT, to help low-income families learn English. I have also been involved with the girls' school at St. Mary's Church and the Chamber of Commerce. I have volunteered with children's playgroups and have seen the impact that childcare dollars have on influencing the needy, and helped feed the homeless in local shelters or city vans.

Due to my profession of meeting planning, it is natural for me to be asked to put together events, and I have chaired many. This is an easy way to use my skills to raise money, and I am happy to do so. The effort is small and the rewards are great. I highly recommend finding organizations in your community where you can lend your talents and become actively involved.

LIFE TIP:

Sometimes working, commuting, and caring for the family is all we can manage. But if you are looking for a way to incorporate volunteering into your life, look at your work schedule and family needs, and determine which days or evenings are usually open or where you have some flexibility with timing. Perhaps during your children's afterschool activities? Then search for an organization that performs the type of services that you feel are most needed, and see if you can arrange to spend an hour or more helping in some way. It could be answering phones every Monday night, or registering people at a monthly event. Tell the organization what you

PART THREE

do best, and perhaps they can find a way to benefit from your wisdom. It is unlikely that they will turn you down!

22. Flexibility: Easing into the Later Years

Life is what happens while you are busy making other plans.

— John Lennon

One day you're making plans to go to the prom, to go to college, to begin a career, to get married, to have a baby, to go on vacation, to write a book. Then all of a sudden you sense that you have more life behind you than you have before you. Plans were made, the actions taken, and you realize that "life" was happening the whole time you were "preparing." Turning the calendar page took just a moment, and the years zoomed by with nary a sound.

And then it hits you like a bucket of cold water in the face. Mortality. You realize that what's in front of you might not be as fun as what is behind you. It's a chore, it's old age—it's what you have to do, not necessarily what you want to do. You start getting the phone calls about your friends or family members that are ill or divorced. Kids are in accidents. Friends die. You start reading the obituaries as often as you used to read your horoscope. You have to pull yourself up and get on with the day, get on with the plans. Keep going through the motions.

But with the work of building your career and raising your family done or almost done, it suddenly becomes clear that you have more free time on

PART THREE

your hands. Now, later in life, you reach out to your friends who are meaningful to you and have nice conversations, impromptu dinners, and relaxing bike rides. It's easy, or at least it seems easy compared to those earlier years when every moment had to be productive. We've done the work! And that's valuable—the life we built—and we cherish the memories and thank God for the times that we treasure behind us. And then life comes full circle, as the younger people in your family are making their way in life, making their plans, getting the jobs, and getting married.

John and I have attended quite a few weddings in recent years, including five in the same year. Five! Three of the couples were in their 20s. The other newlyweds were in their 60s, and those two weddings were very happy occasions. There is new life in the last chapter of your life, and as one of my friends says, "You see life through new glasses." You hear songs in a different way, you experience situations in a different light, wildlife seems more precious, and the love of your family is more valuable than ever. But the plans have changed—you are no longer "building" a life, you are living it! And as they say in AA, just take one step, one day at a time.

In my younger days, I was very determined and had certain goals for my education and career. I was successful. But when I found balance later staying home with my children, it was a spiritual time for me, mostly due to the influence of my children and what I had learned in AA. I had to switch gears and be open to the universe and let go of control. It was much easier to "let go, let God" than I had thought. For the first time in my life, I was letting the day direct me instead of me directing the day. I believe if everyone could take an AA course, the world would be a better place.

If I could live my life over again, I would stop and smell the roses and peonies more in my 20s and 30s, and maybe do less ironing. I would take time to meditate and appreciate the good days. Having positive energy is even more important in this latter stage of life. I want to spend time with people who want to have fun, I want to go to the theater, try new restaurants, and travel. I want to continue learning!

Heading into my late 60s now, it is interesting to look back and analyze the various stages of my life—the paths taken, the choices made, the decisions worth remembering or forgetting. I consider my life to have four distinct chapters. The first was growing up, forming friendships, and learning how I felt about outside influences. The second chapter was discovering my unique skills, putting them to work, and managing my career. During the third stage, I was creating a new life with a partner in marriage, maneuvering my way through motherhood. And now, in the fourth chapter of my life, I am planning for the late years of my life with John, and refining what I have learned and experienced over the years, sharing these lessons whenever possible.

Having completely embraced each stage of my life, I am now embracing this one. I can speak with confidence as I tell you that we can't plan everything in life. Oh, we can have a plan, alright, but we must be willing to stray from it at a moment's notice. We must be open to meeting new people—even if it's a coworker's neighbor who is about to move away. We must consider having new experiences—even if it's learning how to fingerpaint along with your grandchildren. We must stop, look, and listen for opportunity and expect good things to come our way. Be positive about the changes, because more than likely we will learn from them when we are positive. That's the way the universe works.

LIFE TIP:

If you are an American woman approaching your 60s, you most likely have done some analyzing about your life as well. Give some thought to how you want to structure your days. Maybe you are interested in volunteering for a mission trip to help transform lives in another part of the world. Would you like to take a class that you've been putting off for a long time? Basket weaving is still hip, I hear. Do you want to travel someplace exotic or to a neighboring state? Have you seen the USA in your Chevrolet? If not, make some new plans. Go alone, go with a friend, or go with a group. Life is not over just because we're over the hill! Have a new adventure whether it's in your own backyard or a new destination. Explore, be thankful for each day, and continue searching for ways to feel happy, healthy, and whole!

About the Author

Caren Camp currently lives in Alexandria, Virginia with her husband John. Caren started her career in New York City in the fashion industry working for Lilly Pulitzer, Jaeger of London, and Estée Lauder cosmetics. Caren has lived in Charlottesville, Virginia; Los Angeles, California; North Carolina and Northern Virginia for the past thirty years. After staying home for eleven years to raise two boys she decided to get back into work and joined HelmsBriscoe in the meeting planning industry. Caren has been a recovering alcoholic for thirty two years and has learned valuable information by being part of Alcoholics Anonymous. Over the course of her life she has lived in many places, and has worked in a number of industries. She and her husband adopted their two boys. Caren wrote this book to share life experiences which were difficult and yet rewarding, so that it might be easier for others who are facing similar challenges.

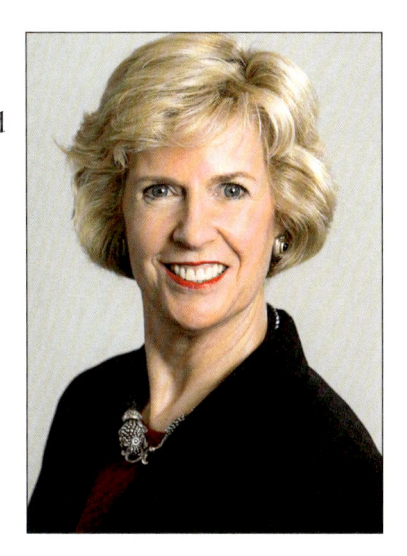